IMPROVING ON PRITIKIN—YOU CAN DO BETTER!

Ross Horne

By the same author
Beat Heart Disease — *1975*
Let's Live A Lot — *1977*
Health Facts Prove The Pritikin Program — *1980*
The Health Revolution 1st Edition — *1980*
2nd Edition — *1983*
3rd Edition — *1984*
4th Edition — *1985*
The Health Revolution Cookbook — *1983*
The Anti-Cancer, Anti-Heart Attack Cookbook — *1984*

ISBN 0 959 4423 9 1

Published by Happy Landings Pty Ltd
P.O. Box 277 Avalon Beach
NSW Australia

Printed by Southwood Press Pty Ltd
80-92 Chapel Street
Marrickville N.S.W. Australia

Contents

Author's Preface

Eleven years ago I was Nathan Pritikin's best disciple and staunchest supporter.

I had observed the Pritikin diet achieve what appeared to be absolute miracles in restoring people who were literally dying back to good health, my own wife being one of them.

Today I still firmly believe in the principles to which Nathan Pritikin devoted the last twenty seven years of his life but I have discovered that the Pritikin diet is far from the best way of implementing those principles.

I have discovered that the beneficial effects of the diet which permit ailing bodies to make rapid recoveries from a great number of complaints, are often accompanied by harmful effects which are subtle enough not to be always noticeably evident, at least not straight away.

Over the years I have observed various manifestations of distress occurring to adherents to the Pritikin diet (myself being one of them) that caused me concern enough to re-write and add one hundred pages to *The Health Revolution* which in its first edition (1981) was Pritikin straight down the line.

Acidosis, arthritis, hypoglycemia, skin and blood disorders were the symptoms I had observed at first, but when cancer started to appear among long-term Pritikin devotees, many of whom I had introduced to the Pritikin diet in the first place, I felt I must make a special effort to point out the potential dangers of all diets which contain large quantities of grain products.

Hence this new volume providing information supplementary to *The Health Revolution,* not only in respect of problems associated with grain products, but also to highlight the faults in the conventional theories of nutrition and to highlight also the fearful dangers presented by our drug-orientated and dismally ineffectual medical system. The inclusion of simple explanations for the so-called "incurable" diseases of civilization, particularly cancer, heart disease, AIDS, arthritis and the common cold, is intended not only to demonstrate the ignorance and confusion existing within the ranks of so-called "scientific" modern medicine, but also to allay the widespread, unnecessary fear associated with these so easily avoided afflictions.

Strong statements such as I have made in this book and in *The Health Revolution* need strong support, and this support is well supplied, particularly by the contributions of Dr Dean Burk of Washington who provided the foreword for *The Health Revolution*, and by Dr Robert Mendelsohn whose opinions on modern medicine appear in chapter nine. Thank you, gentlemen.

In regard to my criticism of the Pritikin diet in the chapters which follow, I wish to make it very clear, here at the beginning, that despite our differences in opinion, my gratitude and respect for Nathan Pritikin, the man, remain undiminished. In my eyes, Pritikin still stands as one of the great Americans of the 20th Century.

And speaking of great men, one who has, in my opinion, done more to advance the knowledge of nutrition than any other single individual, is Dr Edward Howell, formerly of Chicago and now of Fort Myers, Florida. Without the information his research has revealed about natural food enzymes, a proper understanding of the relationship between nutrition and health would be quite impossible. In recognition of Dr Howell's life's work I have dedicated this book to him.

Nutrition, it must be understood, is the sustaining factor of all life, and unless its nutrition is right, no living creature can perform mentally or physically to its true potential in unfaltering health. Society has been on the skids long enough — "health" care and crime bleed away too much of our resources, and bigger and better hospitals and jails are not the answer. Better nutrition must precede better morals and better health.

Dr G. T. Wrench of England illustrated this argument fifty years ago in his wonderful book *The Wheel of Health* in which he offered this advice:

"For progress, therefore, we now have to look backwards. We have raced forward at too great a speed. We have to look back to a period and type of agriculture in which vegetable and animal life were mutually healthy. We have to believe even in the golden age, in which gold did not mean coin in the pocket or blocks in a bank, but an age when the golden sunlight seemed to enter into man through plant and fruit, and bestow the warm gift of health — such an age as the elder Pliny thought upon when he said that for six centuries the men of Rome had needed no physicians."

Happy landings,

Ross Horne
February 1988

Acknowledgements

Modern man has greater knowledge and farther horizons than his predecessors. As each new generation faces the world, the inventors and creators enthusiastically contribute their original ideas to further human progress — often in the face of ridicule, apathy, and stony opposition. The vantage point from which we now survey the world is the product over many centuries, of such men.

To Dr. Edward Howell
with thanks

"*There is little question any more that artery plaque reversal can for the first time be considered possible.*" Dr. Nash in *Circulation,* official journal of the American Heart Association, September 1977.

"*With a cholesterol level of 150 or less, plaque reversal in two years is possible.*" Dr. R. Wissler, Chicago Medical School, addressing the American Heart Association, June 1977.

"*The three major killers in modern society, Coronary Heart Disease, Cancer and Strokes, can all be linked to what people eat and drink.*"Dr. B. Hetzel, Chief of the C.S.I.R.O. Division of Human Nutrition and Foundation Professor of Social and Preventive Medicine, Monash University.

"*The major cancers of our time are diet-caused, mainly by fat and cholesterol.*" Dr. Ernst Wynder, American Health Foundation, addresing the U.S.A. Government Senate Select Committee on Nutrition and Human Needs.

"*With this kind of approach, diet only, 80% of diabetics in this country could be normal in 30 to 90 days.*" Dr. James Anderson, University of Kentucky Medical Centre.

Foreword

to The Health Revolution

by Dr. Dean Burk

(A foundation member of the U.S. National Cancer Institute and former head of the Institute's Cytochemistry Department, Dr. Burk is best known for his work in cancer research for which he has received honors from France, Britain, Germany and the U.S.S.R. Formerly Associate Professor of Biochemistry, Cornell University, he has worked in cancer research at the Kaiser Wilhelm Institute in Germany and at the U.S.S.R. Academy of Science, Moscow. Dr. Burk is the recipient of the Domagk Prize for cancer research, a Knight Commander of the Medical Order of Bethlehem, and a Knight of the Mark Twain Society. He is co-author of the books Cancer, Approaches to Tumor Chemotherapy *and* Cell Chemistry, *and author of over 250 published scientific papers.)*

Having spent most of my professional life in the field of cancer research — a field of great complexity and no little confusion — I was astonished and delighted to become acquainted with this book.

My astonishment arises from the discovery that a layman (the author is a retired airline captain) should have gained such a comprehensive understanding of the complex biological processes which lead to the disease called cancer and to be able to describe these processes in a manner easily understandable by other laymen.

The author describes the origins of not only cancer but of other so-called diseases of civilization and the natural measures required to avoid and control them.

When it is considered that few medical professionals possess this knowledge, this is no mean achievement . . .

The strength, integrity and happiness of a nation are directly proportional to the state of health of its citizens. In the distant past civilizations have risen, flourished and declined, their ruins covered by desert sands. Did affluence destroy them? Are we heading the same way?

Perhaps humans are too clever for their own good. In the pursuit of progress and pleasure they at the same time sow the seeds of their own destruction.

Modern man must comprehend the message presented in this book that the greatest threat to his survival is not that of nuclear war, because although that threat is real, at least everyone is aware of it. The threat most dangerous to mankind comes from the destroyers active right now, subtle and unseen — the poisoning of our soil and water supplies, the de-naturing of our food, the ever-increasing destruction of the environment.

No more do people die of old age — instead, heart attacks, strokes, cancer, diabetes and so on, are today accepted as normal causes of death. Influenza, arthritis, indigestion, constipation, aches and pains and medicine, are a normal part of life. Are coronary bypasses, hysterectomies, reading glasses, hearing aids, wheelchairs, false teeth and plastic hip joints, to be considered normal too?

On his long evolutionary journey, man has strayed onto dangerous ground. Now we are at a crossroads, and whichever way we take there will be some rough going. As ever, the fittest will survive.

Ross Horne's book is a survival manual for the trip ahead.

Dean Burk
Washington D.C.

Foreword 2

by Dr. Ruth Cilento M.B.B.S. D.B.M.

Since 1983 I have led the Quality of Life Group for people with cancer and their families. We used to meet then at the Relaxation Center in Brisbane and it was there that Ross Horne came to lecture us while touring the country for the promotion of his Anti-Cancer, Anti-Heart Attack Cookbook.

Not having read any of his books, I thought at the time he was a fanatic, his ideas unfounded. However, because we were both pursuing the same line of enquiry — the nutritional basis of health and disease — I finally put aside my prejudice and read "The Health Revolution". I was most impressed by the book and realized the tremendous amount of research that had gone into the formulation of Ross's ideas.

Nathan Pritikin's own story, related in "The Pritikin Program", convinced me further to examine his therapy in the treatment of my patients with heart disease, other vascular diseases, and obesity. Following some successes with these patients, I joined the Pritikin Association in 1985 and since then have lectured to many interested groups on how the Pritikin Program works to restore health.

In relation to developing my nutritional therapy for cancer, in 1984 I visited the Hippocrates Center in San Diego, California, and observed there that the raw food diet advocated by Ann Wigmore coincided very much with the concepts Ross had put forward at the Relaxation Center in 1983.

When later reviewing the results of my cancer patients' different dietary programs, I realized that none of the patients on the strict Pritikin Program were recovering, but some others on the Gerson system, the Raw Food diet or my Cilento Way, were keeping their cancers at bay.

Although there are minor differences, what these last three dietary programs have in common is the severity of their restrictions and **each diet is based on a preponderance of raw, fresh, preferably organically grown, fruit and vegetables.** The restrictions prohibit food processed, refined, canned, packaged, smoked, heat dried, chemically treated, colored, flavored or preserved, irradiated, fried or microwaved. Prohibited also are salt, condiments, extracted sugars, extracted oils, hard animal fat, tea, coffee, cola, alcohol or other stimulating drinks. Water must be free of chemicals. Tobacco, marihuana and other toxic substances are forbidden.

These guidelines are stricter in some respects to those of the Pritikin Program, which, diet-wise, could be interpreted as providing a big preponderance of cooked grains and vegetables.

Ross believes that the cooking of food is an unnatural process, damaging to the nutritional value of the food, and in the long run damaging to the people who eat the food, as he has explained so ably in his books and substantiated in his own case studies. Going further, his research and keen observations have led him to believe that grains may be one of the culprits in setting the stage for cancer.

In my nutrition and stress control medical practise I have found that many people do have allergies to grains and grain products and I think it is logical to assume that many others may be adversely affected by these foods without however displaying obvious symptoms. Apart from the objections held by Ross against grains generally, a further objection must be the multitude of chemicals used today in their production, some of which chemicals become residual to a greater or lesser extent in the final food products.

In the light of the fact that degenerative diseases are becoming more widespread, even among the young, and that cancer is now the second commonest cause of death in our society, the observations Ross has made must be taken very seriously indeed. It is my hope that this book will stimulate concerned people to facilitate more research into the potential of improved dietary correction in the prevention and reversal of disease, particularly in view of the fact the benefits are so easily demonstrable, while on the other hand, conventional methods continue to be disappointing.

Ruth Cilento
April 1988

"Sit down before fact as a child.
Be prepared to give up every pre-conceived notion. Follow humbly where nature leads, or you will learn nothing."

Thomas Huxley

Introduction

Nathan Pritikin was a self-trained, highly successful electronics engineer and inventor who, when his life was threatened at age 42 by severe coronary heart disease and leukemia, became a self-trained nutritionist in an attempt to survive. With the development of the diet that bears his name, he not only succeeded in completely reversing his heart disease and stabilizing his blood condition when all the doctors and nutritionists said it could not be done, but he achieved as well something even harder — he forced the medical establishment to accept the fact that it was all possible.

Pritikin demolished a lot of medical dogma and a lot of nutritional dogma too, by demonstrating that they were false, and by demonstrating that his ideas were better and they worked.

But because a system works does not necessarily mean that it is ideal, and we must be careful, when accepting new ideas, not to substitute one lot of dogma for another.

Like Nathan Pritikin and many other people, the writer's interest in nutrition began when a threat presented itself. I was lucky, the warning was early — just a touch of arthritis at age 36. The doctor said arthritis was a fact of life, and I would have to get used to it. I was disappointed with this advice and decided to enquire further into the subject.

Not long after that, on duty as a Qantas pilot I was passing through Singapore; we used to stay at the old Raffles Hotel where I would have scrambled eggs for breakfast and read the *Straits Times*. This day in 1961 there was in the paper an article by Lelord Kordel about nutrition and health, and as I read it I suddenly realized there was a way to get rid of arthritis. I started reading all the books on nutrition I could get.

My studies continued. I ate less meat, ate more fruit and vegetables, and the arthritis went away. And that's how an airline pilot started in the field of nutrition.

While all this was going on, little did I know Nathan Pritikin in Santa Barbara, California, was busy developing a dietary program for the reversal of coronary heart disease, and little did we both know that the concepts we were each evolving applied to the removal of all diseases, not only heart disease and arthritis, and that the same concepts had been all worked out long before by others like us in previous generations.

Heart disease I took only a fairly casual interest in until in 1966 a couple of surprising events occurred suddenly. Two of my contemporaries, both captains on Boeing 707s in Qantas, had heart attacks. They were both 42 years old — same age as me. Like all pilots, they had had medical checks twice a year all their adult lives; they were healthy, swam, played golf — but there they were, grounded with heart disease.

Napoleon once said: "There are two levers for moving men — interest and fear." I would venture the opinion that the most effective lever of the two would be fear, so with increased interest and a touch of fear, my study of the subject of heart disease intensified.

At this time I still believed in the myth of a high protein diet, much of which protein I obtained from muesli, wholewheat products etc., and firmly believed also in the virtues of polyunsaturated oils and margarine — a dietary program similar to that still followed today by many health conscious people.

At age 45 I was smitten by the 'aerobics' bug. I conscientiously ran the parks and roads of the various cities where Qantas crews laid-over. Time of day did not matter, nor did snow or heat or rain, and many were the funny stories that circulated about my peculiar habits. I have been halted by armed guards, bushed in jungles, chased by dogs, and threatened by motorists. I was very fit, never 'caught cold', could 'party on' with the best of them, and in fact never missed a flight with sickness in thirty four years. I thought I knew all about cholesterol, triglycerides and blood viscosity and how to avoid heart disease, and so wrote a small book which was produced by the Qantas publication section called *Beat Heart Disease.*

My wife and I had separated some years before but I looked after her and provided her with a house not far away. I was concerned about her because her diet was bad; she smoked and got little exercise. Eventually in 1975 the heart attack I had predicted occurred; it was massive and she hovered between life and death for weeks. Fortunately I convinced her not to eat the hospital food and she was sustained mainly by the fresh carrot and apple juice I brought in to her each day.

Those people who have read *The Health Revolution* will know this story, so I shall be brief. Without any instruction about diet, exercise or smoking, she was eventually sent home. I carefully supervised her diet, making sure she used polyunsaturated margarine and vegetable oil as recommended by the National Heart Foundation. How was I to know that Dr Meyer Friedman of San Francisco had in 1965, in the Journal of the American Medical Association, reported the devastating effects of such fats in sticking blood cells and platelets together? No wonder she kept on having angina attacks and repeated excursions into intensive care!

Over in California Nathan Pritikin's ideas by this time had paid off. He had demonstrated himself to be completely free of heart disease and had further demonstrated at the War Veterans' Hospital in Los Angeles that he had achieved the same results with 'cardiac cripples' he had worked with there. He was invited to present a paper on the subject of rehabilitation of heart patients at a medical conference in Atlanta, Georgia. This was the 51st Annual Session of the Congress of Rehabilitation Medicine and the 37th Assembly of the Academy of Physical Medicine and Rehabilitation in November 1975. It was the first time a non-medical person had presented a paper at such a conference, but Pritikin's presentation was so successful that the story was reported around the world, and I read about it in the Sydney *Sun* a few days later. The report described the dramatic improvements of elderly heart patients when placed on a program of diet and exercise (the Pritikin Program), and because I thought I knew it all, I read it too quickly, an error which nearly killed my wife.

In and out of hospital Joan went, and I knew that this sequence could end only in one way, so I arranged an angiogram for her with the chief of cardiothoracic surgery at Prince Henry Hospital with a view to bypass surgery. The test revealed two main coronary arteries totally blocked and the third partly so with an aneurism. She was beyond surgery and in a dying condition, said the cardiologists.

It was at that time something made me re-read the newspaper report and suddenly I realized my dreadful mistake, because in the report it clearly stated that *all* fats must be removed from the diet — *including those unsaturated and polyunsaturated.* The news article had not even mentioned Pritikin's name, no one had ever heard of him before. I straight away put an urgent call through to Santa Barbara without even knowing the number and that's how I first met Nathan Pritikin, who quickly and calmly verified my mistake and predicted confidently that Joan would survive. I remember his exact words: "We can help you, we have had a great deal of success with people in that condition." I could tell by his voice he knew what he was about. As soon as we had finished talking I got in my car and proceeded directly to the hospital, where fortunately I knew Professor Wilcken who was in charge of the coronary ward and was able to straight away arrange the special diet needed, which of course was a very simple one. That was in 1976, and as described in *The Health Revolution,* she was mobile again in three days and remains alive and kicking still today despite her occasional lapses in the program.

Joan is only one of thousands of similar cases. So you can see why it is so easy to accept the Pritikin diet as maybe the best in the world.

In 1977 I retired from Qantas and started writing *The Health Revolution* to tell the Pritikin story. I attended all the Pritikin conferences and was appointed the official representative for Nathan Pritikin in Australia. Copies of the Pritikin research data I sent to the Federal and State Ministers for health, to many prominent cardiologists and civic dignitaries, all of whom ignored it, which made me realize the importance of making my book a success.

Nathan Pritikin gave me much information and personal advice and even read carefully through my manuscript to make sure it was right. I was his most ardent disciple and of course followed the Pritikin Program to the letter. *The Health Revolution* was an instant best seller when it was released in Australia and, content with my success, I anticipated being able at last to get some work done on my vintage cars.

This was not to be, because a lot more interesting things were about to happen, some of which were very disturbing . . .

CHAPTER ONE

Second Thoughts On The Pritikin Diet

When Nathan Pritikin began experimenting with diet he did so with one single great purpose in mind, and that was to reverse the disease blocking his coronary arteries. In 1958 coronary bypass surgery was not available to him and it was a matter of either accepting the medical prognosis of an early death from heart failure, or finding a way out for himself. He decided to try diet.

The medical experts said it could not be done and so did the nutrition experts, but Pritikin, having studied all the medical research information, knew that animal experiments had not only proven it was bad diet which caused arteries to block but also that a proper diet allowed blocked arteries to clear again. The experiments with monkeys by Dr Jeremiah Stamler had been most revealing because, physiologically, the body systems of monkeys are almost identical with those of humans, and they work in precisely the same way. When monkeys were fed diets high in fat, cholesterol and protein, their arteries became choked with fatty deposits and cholesterol, and if they were then fed food low in fat, cholesterol and protein, their arteries gradually became clean and healthy again.

Another thing Pritikin knew from experimental evidence of a grimmer nature was that in the German concentration camps during World War II, autopsies on the bodies of dead prisoners showed that after a while on the starvation diet fed to them, no sign of artery disease could be found anywhere in their bodies.

Pritikin knew it was the conventional American diet, high in fat, cholesterol and protein that had caused his heart disease, and he knew that studies of primitive natives in Africa revealed that heart disease and most other diseases of civilization were unknown among them. The diet of these natives was almost entirely vegetarian, very low in fat, consisting largely of corn, vegetables and fruit, and so it was this 'primitive African diet' that Pritikin used as a model for his proposed new Pritikin diet. As Pritikin used to say, he invented nothing new — he merely took an existing diet and adapted it to suit American tastes.

Pritikin aimed first and foremost to lower the levels of cholesterol and fat in his blood because these were the two most dangerous dietary factors contained in the 'normal' American diet. He knew too that his previous diet had contained far too much protein, and because all of these harmful substances are contained in large amounts in foods of animal origin, it meant that his new diet must be almost totally vegetarian and consist of foods mainly of a carbohydrate nature.

Pritikin proceeded with extreme caution because all the so-called experts predicted he would perish from malnutrition, but as he made his dietary changes, one by one, his blood tests showed that the animal tests were exactly predictive of his progress, and this gave him the confidence to more quickly complete his dietary changeover.

By dietary change alone Pritikin reduced his blood cholesterol reading from 280 mg% to 110 (7.2 to 2.8 mm/L), an achievement still considered impossible by most doctors today. (News does not spread fast in medical circles.)

In his final analysis, Pritikin specified that the diet should contain, as a percentage of total calories, no more than 10% fat, 10% protein, and the remaining 80% to consist of complex carbohydrate foods mainly in the form of grain products. Fruit he limited to four pieces per day because he thought the sugar in fruit would raise blood triglyceride levels.*

Pritikin then embarked on an exercise program based on the aerobic exercise concept because he knew also from experimental animal data that exercise promoted blood circulation and helped to clean the arteries. After several years of physical training Pritikin felt he had succeeded in his mission; he could run seven miles with no sign of distress, whereas at the beginning of his program he was incapable of walking the length of a city block.

At the beginning of his program his stress ECG had shown serious heart malfunction at a heart rate of only 80 beats a minute, but in 1966 at the University of California he demonstrated his renewed body by running on the treadmill for 20 minutes with a heart rate of 177, showing no malfunction whatever. He was not only alive and well, but was one of the fittest men in the USA!

Pritikin opened his Longevity Center in 1976 in Santa Barbara and in 1978 he moved it to Santa Monica where it still is. Research data on many thousands of patients passing through the Center since then show the Pritikin diet to be not only effective against heart and other artery disease but also against diabetes, hypertension and many other symptoms of physical degeneration.

There is no doubt that the lives of many thousands of people have been saved by the Pritikin diet and many more lives restored to happy productivity again. It would certainly appear that Nathan Pritikin's claim of his diet being the best in the world was a justifiable one . . .

In 1980 I completed writing *The Health Revolution.* It was dedicated to Nathan Pritikin and consisted of 300 pages of Pritikin, right down the line. I was sticking rigidly to the Pritikin diet myself and was running six miles every day. At my pilot medical check-ups the doctor said I had the arteries and blood

*As it later became evident, this misconception about fruit was a tragic one because it made necessary the adoption of grain products as the mainstay of the Pritikin diet — see chapter 10.

pressure of a schoolboy, resting pulse rate 42. This was comforting news for a man of 56 and I felt rather smug.

By this time I had been studying the subject of cancer for about a year, it being clear that cancer was yet another disease of civilization related primarily to dietary factors. My practise was to start work in the early morning and work right through until sundown when I would go running to tone myself up. I ate strictly Pritikin — lots of oats for breakfast, Pritikin cookies for snacks, salads with Pritikin wholewheat bread for lunch, and some rice or pasta main course for dinner. I had about six to eight pieces of fruit a day which Pritikin said was acceptable if no triglyceride problem existed.

Repeatedly, however, every afternoon an hour or so after lunch I would feel terribly drowsy and on a number of occasions dropped off to sleep while studying, almost as if I'd been drugged. This was the classic symptom of hypoglycemia, but hypoglycemia was one thing Nathan Pritikin claimed was not possible on his diet, the rationale being that complex carbohydrate foods digested slowly and prevented excursions of blood sugar which are the cause of hypoglycemia. It wasn't fatigue I was suffering, because later in the day I'd go running and feel like a million dollars and often work through to midnight. It was hypoglycemia* all right, and the reason for it became clear enough when I read the research work of Dr David Jenkins of the University of Toronto. Dr Jenkins studied the effects of various foodstuffs on blood-sugar levels, and according to the rate the blood sugar was increased, so a certain food was given a 'glycemic rating'. Glucose, the most rapidly absorbed of all, was rated as 100, and other food items were rated on this scale. A high glycemic rating means that the

*A number of Pritikin's patients reported tiredness during the day to which queries Pritikin would suggest they were not perhaps getting enough sleep, which of course may have been the case, or it may have been hypoglycemia. As is explained later, complex carbohydrates may digest rapidly or slowly, depending on what form they are in when eaten and on how much mastication they have received before being swallowed. When bread is eaten and chewed it mixes well with saliva and is consequently digested rapidly with a consequential surge in blood sugar sufficient to be followed by hypoglycemia. (See also Arthritis, chapters 6, 10.)

food item when eaten tends to boost blood sugar to an unnaturally high level, the effect of which is a subsequent slump accompanied by the symptoms of hypoglycemia. Surprisingly, wholegrain bread rated at 72 — higher than refined sugar which only rated 59.

Another thing began to puzzle me. The arthritis I had completely eliminated twenty years beforehand came back again, just where it had been before — in the right elbow. It wasn't severe, but it was more constant and annoying. I knew grain products were acid forming, but surely they couldn't cause arthritis? Or could they?

Then another disturbing thing — dandruff. My skin tone was okay, but I had dandruff; when I brushed my hair it fell like snow. Why? I wondered.

But what worried me more than anything was a slight bleeding from the rectum, first occasionally and then just about every day, sometimes only a trace, other times more. I had noticed this before once or twice a long time previously and a medical examination revealed a fragile blood vessel which the doctor said now and again would bleed, but not to worry about it. I hadn't experienced this bleeding in years, but now it was becoming regular and more profuse. Could all these grain foods be causing this problem too?

I perused every health and nutrition book I had and found a great deal of evidence to show grain products to be potentially quite harmful. In particular, the books of Dr Emmet Densmore and Dr Charles De Lacy Evans of England, doctors who had spent their entire careers in the study of degenerative diseases, were specifically opposed to the use of cereals as suitable foods in the human diet. More of that later.

So I cut grain products out completely and went on to a diet almost completely of raw fruit. I figured that fruit was a far more natural sort of food than cooked dried seeds anyhow. What happened? In a couple of days the arthritis was gone, I experienced no more hypoglycemia, and in about a week the dandruff cleared. The bleeding diminished and in a few weeks ceased altogether.

This was towards the end of 1981 and I've remained on this diet of mainly raw fruit ever since.

In 1982 I planned with Mr Dick Jamieson, owner of the Weight Watchers' franchise in Australia, to set up a Pritikin Center in Sydney. Jamieson had recovered from a heart attack by the adoption of the Pritikin Program and we were both very keen. We met with Nathan Pritikin in Santa Monica and it was agreed that we would go ahead, with me to set the show up and run it. Nathan required that I should spend four weeks at the Longevity Centre in Santa Monica to observe everything that went on and so I was enrolled shortly afterwards as a 'patient' in one of the regular courses which lasted four weeks.

I had told Nathan that I had adopted a diet of fruit, having stopped eating grain products, and he predicted that such a diet would be insufficient to sustain me for long. I already knew that it would, and so for the entire four weeks I spent at the Longevity Center I consumed nothing but fruit, most of which I bought at the excellent fruit market in nearby Venice. Opting out of the gymnasium with its stationary bicycles and treadmills, I went running instead on the beach for six miles every day. Along with the other people on my course, most of whom had heart problems or some such, I had the prescribed medical checks which gave a cholesterol reading of 130 (3.3) and triglycerides 110 (1.2), perfectly acceptable figures.

The most valuable thing I got out of my stay at Santa Monica was a book I discovered in a bookshop there — a book written by Dr Edward Howell called *The Status of Food Enzymes in Digestion and Metabolism.* This was the first and only book I had ever seen or heard of that adequately described the importance of living enzymes in uncooked food, and it confirmed a hundred-fold my argument for the raw fruit diet. It was the most important book discovery I have ever made.

Nathan was unimpressed. He said: "Any chemist will tell you that hydrochloric acid destroys enzymes and that's what happens when raw food enters the stomach, so what does it matter if you destroy them by cooking anyhow?"

If only I could have got him to read Dr Howell's book, what a difference it could have made in his continuing struggle to survive. But I had no idea he had lymphoma and anemia which are diseases of the blood, and I used to put his pasty color down to the fact he worked such long hours indoors all the time under artificial light, in an office without windows. I used to say to him to get out in the sun, but I think most of the time he was just too busy to pay much attention.

Another thing I regretted at the time was the cancellation of a meeting I arranged between Nathan and Charlotte Gerson, daughter of Dr Max Gerson (see chapter 8). Had I known at the time that Nathan suffered from a form of leukemia, I would have arranged again for them to meet, because I knew Charlotte had had quite a lot of success using the Gerson diet in leukemia cases.

I returned home and discussions regarding the new Longevity Center in Sydney were scheduled to continue shortly afterwards when Nathan was due to visit on a lecture tour of Australia.

Not long before Nathan arrived in Sydney I received two interesting phone calls. One was from a fellow who had a couple of years previously cleared his heart and blood pressure problems by going on the Pritikin diet. His first name was Colin and he had phoned me from time to time to report his wonderful progress. I get lots of these reports in letters too. Anyhow, Colin was a bit embarrassed, he said, because when he had first phoned me two years before, he had not mentioned he'd had a prostate problem; he had hoped it would clear up along with his angina etc. But it had not, he said, and it was a constant and great irritation to him. Moreover, he added, a subcutaneous cyst had grown on his back which had had to be surgically removed and so he had come to suspect he was still doing something wrong, what could I suggest? All I could tell him was that Dr Herbert Shelton had said in his books that on a raw vegetarian diet the symptoms of prostate disorder would usually disappear in about seven days. So I suggested to Colin that he go on a raw fruit diet and to see what happened. This he did, and ten days later he phoned again to tell me elatedly that he was free of the symptoms.

The other phone call was from a man in Melbourne who was rather terse. "You say in your book that arthritis is cleared on the Pritikin diet. Well, mine has not; it is getting worse." I had to admit that I had conveyed an erroneous impression in my book's first edition after seeing Jean Halewyn's recovery from severe rheumatoid arthritis, but that was before my own arthritis had come back. So I gave him the advice to abandon cereals and eat raw fruit, explaining my reasons, and he said he would try this.

Two weeks later I was in Melbourne with Nathan Pritikin in my capacity as his aide. My job was to introduce Nathan to the audiences wherever we went and then sit down. The halls were always packed out and although I'd heard it all before, I always found his lectures interesting. At question time someone asked about arthritis and Nathan replied: "We don't do so well with that."

Nathan had a good sense of humor; someone asked him about the gadgets available from which you could hang upside-down suspended by your ankles, supposedly to improve the circulation in some way. Nathan paused for a moment and then replied: "All I can say is that it's a lot better for you than hanging by your neck!"

Anyhow, when the lecture finished and most of the audience headed for the door, the usual enthusiasts headed for the dais to ask more questions. Nathan was surrounded by a big group and I was surrounded by a small group. A middle-aged man approached me, hand outstretched, and as I shook it I said: "What can I do for you?" He replied: "Nothing, you have already done it. I'm the man who phoned you two weeks ago about my arthritis and I just want to tell you it worked."*

*As explained in *The Health Revolution*, there are two main causes of arthritis — high uric acid levels in the blood and high fat levels in the blood. The fat problem is resolved on the Pritikin diet but when too many cereal (grain) products are consumed, particularly bread, the acid problem is exacerbated.

For a number of reasons the proposed Pritikin Center in Sydney did not go ahead, one of them being that I could no longer agree to following the strict Pritikin dietary protocols which, I was convinced, were doing harm along with the undoubted good.

I kept persisting with my argument against the emphasis on cereal foods whenever I met up with Nathan and finally got him to accept a copy of Dr Howell's book, by describing to him how the human pancreas becomes abnormally enlarged by overwork, particularly the overwork of digesting grain products. He took the book but I doubt if he ever read it because he never made any comments. I was so disappointed; this was the book that Professor Geoffrey Bland, the biochemist of international renown had described as most exciting.

Nathan Pritikin's war against fat and cholesterol continued, as so it should have done, but he never ever got to understand that it was the adipose lipase and other enzymes in the raw fatty diet of Eskimos that accounted for their surprisingly low blood cholesterol levels. Had he comprehended that, a lot of other things would have become clear to him. To prove that the fat of avocadoes did not cause excessive levels of triglycerides in the blood and did not increase red cell and platelet aggregation and blood viscosity when the avocado was eaten raw, I had blood tests done which clearly demonstrated this, but once again Nathan was unimpressed, so I gave up trying to influence him.

In the third edition of *The Health Revolution,* now increased to 400 pages, I virtually divorced myself from the Pritikin diet and explained the reason why in great detail.

There I was content to let matters rest; after all, on the Pritikin diet people were in a vastly improved situation anyway and no doubt not many would convert to a completely raw food diet just to get rid of a touch of arthritis.

In 1983 Australia won the America's Cup yachting series at Newport, Long Island, and the most popular hero of the event was Ben Lexcen, designer of the Australian yacht. Hopes for a successful 1987 defense of the Cup rested of course again on Ben and I was disturbed in mid 1984 to read in the news that he was in intensive care with heart disease. So to cut a long story short, I delivered to him a copy of *The Health Revolution,* assuring him if he followed its advice he could reverse his circulatory problems. The next day I left Sydney to go to a conference in Los Angeles and was away about a week. On my return there was a message to call Ben Lexcen, which I did. His wife Yvonne answered the phone and told me Ben was out sailing on the harbour (not bad for a man only a week out of intensive care), but it was not Ben who now had a problem, it was her. She had elected to go on the Pritikin diet and after only a few days had very painful arthritis in her hands.

When people go on the Pritikin diet they feel hungry all the time, and in an effort to satisfy their hunger, and being limited on the amount of fruit they are permitted, they fill up on bread and cookies etc. This is what I had done, so I said to her: "I bet you are eating a lot of bread," to which she replied: "Yes, because I'm hungry all the time and wholegrain bread is legal." So I told Yvonne to cut out the bread and to fill up on fruit, and in a day or two her arthritis was gone. And that's how Ben Lexcen came to write the foreword for Toni Bobbin's *Anti-Cancer, Anti-Heart Attack Cookbook.* (Unfortunately, Ben didn't stick to the program.)

Chapter 2 in *The Health Revolution* is entitled 'Living Proof'. It contains testimonial letters from people who have made wonderful recoveries, having changed their old eating habits for better ones. Some of these letters are reproduced here in this chapter because they illustrate the benefits that can be expected by sick people who adopt the Pritikin diet. Note carefully the stories of Ted Clifton, Trevor Green and Ron McKimm, because what happened to them later demonstrates that on the Pritikin diet you can get into trouble.

Carefully note also that the recoveries of Pam Pritchard and Peter McLarty from cancer were achieved not on the Pritikin diet but on diets of fruit and vegetables.

Ted Clifton, Journalist and Author, Aged Seventy-Four
"Whilst gardening at home one Saturday in September 1976 I suddenly felt waves of nausea and then collapsed on the grass. I managed to stagger inside and fell on my bed. My wife called the doctor who took one look and sent for the ambulance. I had had a heart attack.

"Lying in intensive care in Royal North Shore Hospital, I was covered with wires and tubes and I could see what looked like TV screens with lights moving across them. Time had no meaning, except I knew Sunday was Fathers' Day and I felt a rush of tears and self pity. After some days I was moved into another ward with three other patients, a taxi owner, an architect and a farmer.

"When I had recovered sufficiently to return home I decided to have a complete check-up at the Aerobics Center. I failed the stress E.C.G. and my blood tests were bad, but whilst there I happened to meet Ross Horne, and this meeting changed my life. Ross spoke convincingly and gave me great encouragement; I decided to follow his advice.

"I adopted the Pritikin diet and commenced a walking program. A friend of Ross, Marlene Pentecost (author of *Cooking For Your Life*) provided my wife with cooking recipes and advice. Ross was my chief instructor who, although a busy man as a senior Qantas pilot, always found time to advise me.

"Since embracing the program I have felt uplifted in spirit and my health has improved steadily. In summer I swim 30 laps of my pool. I have found again the desire to work and help others, I have resumed writing and apart from magazine articles, have just written a book. The book is my life story, and I've called it *Take It Easy.*

Pam Pritchard, Housewife and Businesswoman, Aged Forty-Five
"Dear Ross, I'd like to say how excited I felt after reading your

book. I wish it had been available eighteen months ago when I was so desperately searching for an answer to my illness.

"Briefly, after a number of stressful years, in the early part of 1980 I discovered a lump in my breast. Six months later I had a biopsy, the results which proved to be malignant. Believing cancer to be a fatal disease, I was devastated.

"The following weeks placed me in great turmoil, thinking I had no other choice but surgery. At this time I was living on Magnetic Island and a dear friend gave me two books to read — Edie May's *How I Cured Breast Cancer Naturally* and Max Gerson's *A Cancer Therapy, The Results of Fifty Cases.*

"I started thinking maybe — just maybe — there was an alternative to conventional medicine. In face of opposition from the doctors and my family I decided to pursue the methods outlined in these books. Refusing surgery, I started on a natural raw vegetarian diet, exercising and swimming in the sunlight and fresh air.

"I started feeling better and became aware that my previous eating and living habits had been completely wrong.

"Six months later I returned to my family in Sydney and because of their concern, I had another medical examination. Extensive tests revealed no cancer. Not convinced, the doctors pressed me to have chemotherapy and radiotherapy.

"Feeling confused because of opposition from my family and the medicos to what I knew was right, I was introduced to you at just the right time. You were able to reinforce my convictions and more. Your encouragement and support has been wonderful and I cannot sing your praises enough. I know your book is an answer to all disease and hopefully people like myself will find a new way of life through you.

"Something which could have been devastating has changed my whole way of life for the better. May God bless you and again thank you for your personal help and encouragement. I now run my own business and have never felt better."

Vic Roby, Western Australia

"You may remember my writing to you in January of this year, relating briefly my history as regards my triglycerides and cholesterol levels, and how, since reading your *Health Revolution* book, my triglycerides and cholesterol levels have for the first time in the eight or nine years since I first had them checked (and found them to be raised quite high), been lowered to 'normal', thanks to the Pritikin diet and you. My latest blood test result is even better showing my triglycerides at 1.5 and the cholesterol at 3.6.

"My main reason for writing to you again is to tell you about my Father-in-law who lives in England, he is 58 years old, totally blind and has only one leg (the result of an explosion at age 14). Before Christmas 1982, he wrote to tell us that he was suffering from angina, and then at the end of January 1983, he informed us that because he could now only walk about 20 feet before suffering a severe angina 'attack', and because his general condition had worsened, he would be undergoing a triple by-pass operation on March 11th this year. He was obviously very worried about his prospects, so I talked to him at length on the telephone about the Pritikin diet and also purchased another copy of your *Health Revolution* book and sent it to him.

"On receipt of the book his wife read it to him, and also re-read all the relevant parts on triple by-pass operations etc. He immediately put himself 100% on the diet and exercise plan, and set about curing himself.

"One week before his date for the operation, he was walking all over the place, his angina pains non-existent and he felt so much better all over, and so requested another angiogram which showed his atherosclerosis reversing. The surgeon said he didn't know why this was and also said the condition would probably stop reversing soon and continue deteriorating again. He also said (when told by my Father-in-law about the Pritikn diet being responsible for his getting better) that one should ignore such 'fad diets', and even if somehow the diet did reverse my Father-in'law's condition, he would never be able to walk more than two miles. Well, he's already proved the surgeon wrong on that count as well!

"Anyway, the surgeon agreed that the operation no longer appeared necessary and was therefore cancelled; another success for the Pritikin diet.

"I got into conversation with a stranger in my local library some time in January; he was due to have his gallstones removed and was searching for a suitable diet to go on after the operation, but after introducing him to your book, he took my name and 'phone number and off he went, proclaiming that he was going to tell his doctor that he would not be having the operation until he had given the Pritikin diet a chance first.

"Two weeks ago, I received a telephone call from him informing me that he didn't have the operation, and a subsequent examination and tests have shown that his gallstones have almost completely dissolved.

"A lady friend of my wife has, since the age of puberty, experienced a heavy loss of blood during her period as well as premenstrual tension, but since going about 80% on the diet, she experiences no premenstrual tension and hardly any blood loss.

"After previously attempting to ridicule me because of my weight loss workmates are now beginning to realize that what I have been telling them recently makes sense. In fact, now six are 100% on the diet and about another eight are partly on it, which probably explains why none of the Perth or suburban book shops have any copies, or can't obtain any copies of the *Health Revolution,* and also most libraries have a waiting list for it.

"I don't know if you are aware of it or not but on April 3rd, 1983, in Western Australia's *Sunday Independent,* there appeared an article about a man named Graeme Prosser who had cancer of the prostate and a tumor covering the lower third of his bladder. The article mentioned Mr Prosser reading your book and now, after he and his family followed its strict guidelines, it described how his monthly biopsy finds him completely free from cancer.

"Congratulations, Ross!"

'The Miracle of Nature Cure' — Newsletter of the Natural Health Society of South Australia
The following is a case history of NHS member, Trevor Green of Sydney. It is so wonderful that the message must be broadcast loud and clear!

"Eighteen months ago I received the news that I had triple artery disease — right descending artery blocked, left descending artery 70% closed, and the third smaller artery 30% closed. The surgeon I was consulting confirmed that open heart surgery was desirable and that if I did not have it the chances of having a third heart attack were real in the next five years and that it could be fatal. At that time I had just heard about the Pritikin Program which is as you know, a health program similar to the ideals of NHS with the exception of oils and fats not being part of the diet. I had read Ross Horne's book, *The Health Revolution*, with great interest because he had made the statement in the book that if a person followed the regression diet (stricter version) for two years, arteries of the heart would be largely cleared of lesions. The surgeon politely ridiculed this concept when I discussed it with him and replied to my cardiologist that 'I had vocalized false expectations' as to diet.

"All this was a tremendous shock to me. I wrote to Ross Horne who replied simply that if I followed the diet assiduously 'I would not need an operation'. The problem was whether to be safe, as it were, and have the operation, or take a chance for the two years and see if the diet would work. I am now half way through the two year test period and my cardiologist can see that I am doing well under the diet, though he is reserved about its ability to regress heart lesions once formed.

"Unexpectedly, he wrote to me about going into the Prince Alfred Hospital as part of a research program. This involved a two day stay linked up to a heart catheter and an intensive series of exercises, some under certain drugs, some without. I must add I was somewhat apprehensive about having tests which contained a risk factor since you are exercised to exhaustion point, and one wonders just how much exhaustion a defective heart can take! However, I went in with the hope that my contribution might be helpful to somebody else and consoled myself with the expressed sentiments of the hospital cardiologist that 'if anything goes wrong I know what to do!'

"Well, I can tell you with much gladness that not only was I an ideal guinea pig for the purpose of the research project, but also that my heart performance was considered little short of amazing by the cardiologist. At the conclusion of the two days he said to me — 'we exercised you to exhaustion point (ie, my legs gave out on the cycle machine — a device like a dentist's chair tilted back with pedals at the base where one is strapped in with many wires strapped to the body) and there was no sign of failure in the cardiograph.' He then added words which were music to my ears . . .'If I were you I would not have the operation'. Another matter which caused them surprise during the tests was the high amount of oxygen in the blood — so good was the oxygen level that it showed up on the test equipment that I was being administered oxygen.

"All these marvellous results are due to changing to the natural health regimen, eliminating red meat entirely, and most other meat as well. Of course, I have a long, long way to go yet, but the balance between the need for surgery is now on the negative side and this in only twelve months of application, though I must say, assiduous application. A much more telling result will be when I have a second angiogram — dye released into the heart arteries which is then photographed and shows precisely the position and extent of blockages. This will be in about one year's time. My cardiologist says if there is any significant result he will write it up in the Medical Journal."

Roslyn Allen, Schoolteacher, Aged Thirty-Two
Written by her fiance, Sean Hanrahan, Editor, Southern Cross Newspaper, *Victoria.*

"Roslyn became a high school teacher three years ago after working hard at night school to matriculate and then three years of university. Together we drank a bit and generally burned the candle at both ends.

"For some time Roslyn had experienced numbness and tingling in her limbs and at first put it down to the cold weather. These symptoms progressively worsened and were medically diagnosed as multiple sclerosis in December 1980.

"By February the situation was disastrous; she had symptoms everywhere in her body, she was suffering extreme fatigue and depression and she was so tired in the evening she had to go to bed at 6 p.m. The doctors said that nothing could be done and that it may be advisable to move closer to the hospital and to come back whenever it got bad. Expecting to become confined to a wheelchair, she advised me to leave her as she did not wish to be a dead weight in my life.

"About ten weeks ago, dissatisfied with the medical advice, we commenced investigating alternative forms of treatment and read two interesting books on MS — J. C. Ogilvie's *Overcoming Multiple Sclerosis* and W. Richie Russell's *Multiple Sclerosis — Control of the Disease.* Following the dietary advice of the former book, after about two weeks Roslyn started to improve significantly. Then we read your interpretation of the MS process and were so impressed we both immediately adopted the Pritikin Program.

"Roslyn's recovery was noticeably accelerated, and now all symptoms of MS have gone except slightly in her right hand. She looks years younger, and in her own words she has more energy now than ever before in her life; her spirits are soaring.

"For my part I have lost 21 pounds and feel great. We plan to marry at the end of the year."

Elizabeth May Doolin, Pensioner, Aged Seventy-Five

"Dear Captain Horne, I received your last books yesterday and thank you very much for them. I owe you a debt of gratitude for saving my life. I would of been in my grave now if I had not changed doctors and then started on your diet. I was being treated for kidneys.

"In hospital it was a battle to get temperature down. I had convulsions, nose-bleeds etc. When home I was getting worse — could not walk and was not able to stand to press my slacks to go to the doctor. When I complained I was told 'Just sit around in a chair'. Ironing was out. So changed doctor. He took blood tests, ECG, urine test and said it was heart and a pacemaker was needed.

"As I am a war widow I came under Repat and arrangements had to be made. Someone on television recommended a clove of garlic a day as it was a pick-up for the heart, so I started taking it. Then, going through old papers I had kept, came on your *Daily Mirror* writing and so started on the Pritikin diet. It was when I went to the doctor to find out what was to be done about the heart-pacer. When he examined me he said 'There is a change, something is working.' Asked what I had been doing and what medicine. I told him that I was eating garlic every day and about the Pritikin Diet. The doctor said go on as you are going and he would see me in a few days. Next visit he was very pleased but told me not to try and lose weight as the body was too weak.

"He is very pleased with me now. Never had any colds in the winter, can go shopping. Going back every week to the Community Center. Doing most of the cooking for the family, get up at about 8.30 a.m., sometimes earlier. Go all day and as my daughter and husband are cleaners and work at night I cook their tea and am lucky to be in bed by 2 a.m. I walk some distance and know my limits. If I have a busy day I get very tired and make the next day easy.

"My doctor is very interested in the Pritikin diet plan. My

tablets have been cut down and I have not taken garlic for a while. It was a real pick-up for me. It used to make the pulse beat better.

"I am 75 years and feeling well again. I thank you and hope that you will live to enjoy life, also your wife. May God bless you."

Peter McLarty, 39, Managing Director of large engineering company, Western Australia

"On New Year's Eve 1980 I was informed by my family doctor that the blood test I had taken the day before indicated leukemia. Further tests the following day at Royal Perth Hospital confirmed I had Hairy Cell Leukemia and that my spleen was grossly enlarged.

"The medical specialist recommended immediate removal of the spleen as the only course of treatment available for this disease. After considerable discussion and thought I reluctantly agreed, and so the operation was performed on January 8, 1981.

"After the operation blood cell and platelet counts returned to normal but although the Hairy Leukemia Cells were no longer present in the blood, they continued to be numerous in the bone marrow.

"The specialist advised that no more medical treatment existed. His advice was to wait until the Hairy Leukemia Cells overpowered the bone marrow and prevented the production of blood cells, at which stage (in an expected 18-24 months) chemotherapy would be tried. However, he was not optimistic about the chemotherapy as it had always failed in the past. He offered no other advice but he specifically warned against an organic diet as a useless waste of effort because no benefits could be expected from its use.

"As a positive thinker, I refused to accept this attitude; I believed I had caused the problem and I believed therefore that I could fix it.

"I suspected that my condition was a result of unrelenting stress over a long period of time, and this stress, combined with my traditional Australian diet, was perhaps the cause of my problem.

"I immediately began to discover all I could about Hairy Cell Leukemia and began also to be concerned about the overall state of my body. I frequented the medical libraries of local hospitals, I researched all the medical computer data banks and I read every medical article on the disease. At the same time I began to walk ever increasing distances each day.

"Reading the first medical journal article was a traumatic experience. Sitting in the Fremantle Hospital medical library with tears streaming down my face I gained a chilling knowledge of the survival rate for my disease. Chemotherapy was a total failure. Patients were reduced to a series of numbers, their survival time plotted in months, and few months at that.

"Only one medical paper gave a clue that provided encouragement. It was a South African medical journal and it gave the history of one individual patient with Hairy Cell Leukemia who for no apparent reason had, over a number of years, eliminated all signs of the disease.

"This was all the encouragement I needed. If it could happen to that one person, then it would happen for me also.

"A friend introduced me to a Christian Brother who had contracted melanoma seven years earlier. After being told he would survive only a few months, Brother John Mann adopted the strict vegetarian way of life and recovered his health. After hearing his story and speaking with others, I became a strict vegetarian in February 1981.

"I planned my diet methodically. The first stage was to produce a cleansing process to restore my body to an alkaline chemistry condition. For one week I ate grapes only, every two hours during the day. Stage two consisted of vegetable puree every three hours and the third stage, the mainstay of the diet regimen, consisted of fresh salads, almonds and fruit, together with frequent fresh vegetable juices. After a few months I allowed myself some steamed vegetables as well.

"Tests over the next twelve months showed no leukemia cells in the blood, but still signs of them in the bone marrow. However, after fifteen months, a bone marrow test at the M. D. Anderson Hospital, Houston, Texas, showed completely clear.

"Having experienced natural healing for myself, reading books about it and talking with others who have been naturally healed of various complaints, I am convinced that diet is the answer to all modern diseases. Diet combined with a worry-free, relaxed mental state, provides the answer to any chronic medical condition. The problem is our so-called modern society cannot accept something so simple.

"Because other people helped me, I have tried to assist anyone who may be in the state of medical limbo that I experienced. It is difficult for anyone in fair health to adopt the strict vegetarian way of life, even though they may accept the logic of it. But when the time arrives — when they become desperately sick — it is really very easy, and it works.

"IT IS THAT SIMPLE.

"Ross, good luck."

In addition to these 1981 accounts there is the story of Ron McKimm with whom I joined the Royal Australian Air Force in 1942. He became a Spitfire pilot and I became a flying instructor, but after only intermittent contact over the years we met up again in about 1979. He had made a career of the Air Force and had retired with the rank of Air Commodore. I had not long retired from my career as a Qantas pilot and being very fit I was dismayed to find him a 'cardiac cripple', unable to walk up his drive in the morning to get the paper without resting with chest pain. Needless to say I had him on the Pritikin diet straight away, and needless to say, in two weeks he was out playing 72 holes of golf a week with lots of swimming as well. The Brisbane *Sun* newspaper featured a picture of him running on the beach. Great stuff, we couldn't afford to lose McKimm.

1985

Our story now centers on Nathan Pritikin and three of his most devoted and meticulous followers: Ted Clifton, Ron McKimm and Trevor Green, whose stories you have just read.

A beautiful summer's day in Avalon Beach, Sydney. I got in my car to go to the village and on the radio the news was just finishing. I only caught the last of it and thought I was mis-hearing things. Nathan Pritikin dead? Suicide? Cancer? I felt chilled, I couldn't believe it, but it was true. I phoned Nathan's son, Robert, and for the first time found out what Nathan had kept from the world for 27 years; he had had leukemia, Robert said, caused by radiation treatment of some kind back in 1957. Anemia too. Suddenly I realized why his color had been bad and why he worked so frantically on his latest research project. He had felt all along he was on borrowed time. So passed a great man.

But 1985 had other shocks for me. Ted Clifton, my second Pritikin patient of 1976, died. I hadn't even known he'd been sick. It was cancer.

Then my old mate McKimm, in a few months riddled with cancer, died too.

Then a phone call from Trevor Green, probably the best Pritikin success story of them all. This was Trevor's second request for advice, what was it this time? Cancer, he said, an invasive malignant growth on his forehead with others on his back. Should he let them operate? I gave Trevor the same advice as I had in 1981 regarding the bypass surgery but with one major difference. I said why not get off the Pritikin diet and see what happens on the Gerson raw food diet? Two years have passed since then, and Trevor, on the Gerson diet, reports his cancer to be gradually diminishing. (See Update on Trevor Green, end of chapter.)

Now three cases of cancer in a world where cancer abounds would probably not cause a great deal of concern in conventional medical circles, but if the real causes of cancer (see chapter 6) are even remotely understood then these three cases become highly significant.

It is an unquestionable fact that the Pritikin diet has caused arthritis to occur in the bodies of a lot of people, and that the blame for this can be squarely placed on the high consumption of grain products, particularly when not balanced by the intake of sufficient raw vegetables and fruit.

A major anomaly which becomes apparent when the practised Pritikin diet is compared with the original Pritikin guidelines is that the actual protein content of the diet in real life may vary between 12% and 20% of the total calories, which is a great deal higher than the 10% originally recommended. When it is considered that the optimal protein intake for the human body is only three to four per cent, it becomes clear that the Pritikin diet can be so excessive in protein that metabolic upsets must be expected, and premature wear and tear on the body's vital organs becomes inevitable.

Excessive protein is recognised to be a potent cause of cancer. Unfortunately the emphasis of the Pritikin teachings has been almost entirely on the danger of fat and cholesterol, so that the potential of protein to cause harm has gone almost unnoticed.

Whereas arthritis eventuates in the presence of a bloodstream of an acid nature usually associated with a diet high in animal protein and/or fat, a diet high in vegetable protein (and/or vegetable fat) may just as readily produce the same result. Stress, of course, is a well known exacerbating factor.

Now all the dietary factors underlying the development of various forms of arthritis have been shown just as clearly to be associated with the eventual development of various forms of cancer and for that matter most of the other metabolic upsets that plague civilized man. Of course the vitamin and mineral status of a diet also affects the issue, and it is possible that the most potent factor of all may well be the destruction of natural enzymes by the ever-present cooking process.

To put the argument in a nutshell: just as arthritis will never occur in a body furnished with a pure, oxygen-charged bloodstream, nor will healthy tissue cells of the body, in the same favorable circumstances, de-differentiate to become cancer cells.

When arthritis, prostatitis, hypoglycemia, cancer or any other upset occurs in someone's body it is clear that that person's diet errs seriously in one aspect or another. And the truth of this statement is verified by the fact that when the Pritikin diet is abandoned in favor of the Gerson (raw) diet these symptoms of blood disorder quickly begin to diminish.

It is an old saying in medicine that a man is as old as his arteries. But it is a greater truism to say a man is as healthy as his blood.

The Pritikin diet does wonders for the arteries and it unsticks the blood so that it flows easily, but that is not enough. We want the chemistry of our blood to be right. We must improve on Pritikin.

Update on Trevor Green — April 1988

After the initial promising results from his raw food diet, Trevor's cancers stabilized, neither growing nor shrinking, and although he has maintained an otherwise excellent state of health, he had begun to despair of ever ridding himself of them by natural means. Then, only a few weeks ago, listening to a recorded lecture by Charlotte Gerson (see chapter 8) he learned that blood pressure medication was injurious to the liver (as well as causing impotence) so he immediately stopped the medication he had been on for years. Since then Trevor reports a noticeable improvement in his condition and is once again confident of achieving the complete 'spontaneous remission' as demonstrated by others following the Gerson regimen.

CHAPTER TWO

Healthy Blood, Healthy Cells, Healthy Body

"In Nature there are neither rewards nor punishments. . . There are consequences."

Robert Ingersoll

Everyone knows that the body is made up of living cells, billions and billions of them, but few stop to consider that each and every cell of which they are made is, in its own right, an individual living organism. Each cell in fact is a citizen, as it were, of a tightly-knit community. The cell's first concern of course is its own survival, its second concern being its contribution to the best interests of its community of fellow cells.

If each and every cell of the body is well-nourished and healthy then so too will the whole body be healthy.

Examined under a microscope, the cells of different body tissues can be identified as to what kind they are because, according to their function — e.g. lung tissue, skin, bone and so on — they vary in size and structure. Different as they may be, it is an incredible fact that every one of them is a descendant of one parent cell, the fertilized egg cell, which shortly after conception subdivides into two cells, again into four, and so on. As the pregnancy continues, at first the cells of the embryo all look alike; they are 'undifferentiated' and grow rapidly as if out of control. Then, as the embryo grows, the cells start to become different, and so begins the construction of the different organs of the body. This process is called differentiation, and as it continues, each new generation of cells becomes more and more different and specialized and at the same time their growth becomes 'controlled' and slows down, until the foetus is complete, at which stage the cells are said to be fully differentiated.

It is interesting to note that just after conception the undifferentiated embryo cells resemble primitive single-cell life-forms still to be found in the ocean, which reflects the fact that it was from such primitive organisms that higher forms of life evolved. Further demonstrating this evolutionary process is the fact that as the embryo develops, in the early stages it resembles almost exactly the embryos of all the other animals on Earth, even at one stage having gills like a fish, and later, a tail, which features disappear as differentiation proceeds.

Why all this talk about cells? Well, it's simply to emphasize that when we get around to discussing correct nutrition and its relationship with health and long life, it is the nutrition of the cells and the health of the cells that must be considered above all else.

To continue, the nutritional substances and oxygen needed by the cells they take in directly from the fluid environment in which they live, and their waste products are discharged into the same fluid. In this way the highly specialized cells of the human body function still in exactly the same fashion as the primitive single cell creatures which have inhabited the waters of ponds and oceans for a billion years or so. The cells of all animals live like this, using a system Mother Nature invented millions of years ago when the higher forms of life first evolved. With great numbers of cells grouped together they could not all have access to the seawater and the organic nutrients it contained, so a circulatory system had to be provided. And when land creatures first evolved they carried within them their own 'sea' to bathe and nourish their body cells. This fluid is called lymph and flows constantly in the tissues being replenished all the time by fluid from the main bloodstream.

So to have healthy cells it is obvious you must have good quality lymph with lots of oxygen, and to get that it is further obvious that you must in the first place have clean, pure, free flowing blood containing lots of oxygen. To have good blood it is essential then to eat food which provides the nutrients the body needs without at the same time loading it with undesirable substances, even though for a time the digestive organs — liver, kidneys etc. can do a pretty good job of blood purification.

Although all living creatures on Earth vary enormously in shape, size and activity, and their diets vary from totally vegetarian to totally carnivorous, the functions of the cells of their bodies are all much the same and so are the nutritional requirements of the cells. The nutrition of all creatures is provided by plants of one kind or another, the vegetarian animals taking it directly from the plants, and the carnivorous animals indirectly from the prey they eat, which are made of substances they have obtained by eating plants. Although the different diets vary tremendously, the lymph bathing the cells within all these different looking creatures is the same, and this state of affairs is due to the fact that each specie of animal is equipped with a digestive system exactly suited to its natural diet. Thus the long, complicated digestive system of a bullock can break down well chewed grass into the basic nutritional components needed by the cells of its body, while in a less complicated way the short, smooth digestive tract of a dog can break down the flesh of a bullock swallowed in haste, unchewed, to obtain the same nutritional substances which came from grass in the first place.

If an animal is fed a diet unsuited to its digestive system, it may still manage to survive, because the digestive systems of all animals are capable of a certain degree of adaptation, but the animal will not do so well nor will it live as long as it should, because of the undue strain imposed on the vital organs of its body which strive at all times to maintain the quality of the blood. Few humans eat a diet really suited to their digestive systems, and just as the traditional diets of different populations vary widely around the world, so do the disease rates and life-spans vary too, even though, regardless of the diet, good health may prevail in youth when the vital organs remain relatively intact.

Thus, whatever the diet, good or bad, while ever the digestive system, liver, kidneys etc. can produce good blood from it and get rid of impurities to provide pure lymph to bathe the cells, so will the entire body remain in sound health. Once the vital organs degenerate to the point that the purity of the bloodstream is compromised, that is when the symptoms of disease commence to appear. This unhappy situation eventuates usually as middle-age approaches and could well be said to be the actual cause of aging in the first place.

The rate at which old-age and disease displaces youth and vigor depends more than anything else upon the condition in which the bloodstream is maintained, and once the signs of degeneration appear, no medicine on Earth can help. The only course of action possible to arrest the degenerative process is to restore favorable circumstances within the body by reverting to correct diet, the very source of life to the body's cells.

The concept of body health being whole and indivisible — related directly to the quality of the interior fluids, blood and lymph, is one centuries old, but was never entertained seriously within the medical profession until propounded scientifically by the great French physicians Claude Bernard and Antoine Bechamp a little over one hundred years ago. Bernard coined the term *milieu interieur* and insisted that it was only when the *milieu interieur* became defective that microbes could multiply and cause the symptoms of disease in the body, which meant of course that the treatment of any disease should start with the correction of the *milieu interieur.* This concept has been proven over and over and has been demonstrated in Nature for millions of years.

Unfortunately, just as the concept of the *milieu interieur* was gaining acceptance in medical circles, Louis Pasteur came up with his theory that germs were the cause of disease, and his demonstrations with vaccines on animals appeared to dramatically prove the theory. So dramatic in fact were his demonstrations that the germ theory took over the minds of doctors world wide, and there it still resides, as displayed today by the frantic efforts being made to find a vaccine against AIDS, even though it has never been proven that AIDS is anything more than a syndrome, and only apparently related to the so-called AIDS virus. Ironically, Pasteur himself realized the error of his theory before he died and said to his friend Professor A. Renon who was caring for him: "Bernard was right, the microbe is nothing, the soil (*milieu interieur*) is everything."

The difference between the metabolic diseases of degeneration and the various infectious diseases is explained in chapter 6, but the point that Bernard tried to make, and to which Pasteur himself later agreed, was that a vigorously healthy body never displays disease of any kind, whether exposed to germs or not, and that germs (and viruses) are only opportunistic scavengers that take advantage of a weakened organism, and as such cannot be considered the prime cause of any disease.

Animals in the wild are sleek and healthy all through their lives, while humans are constantly affected by some health problem or another. Why do humans live in constant fear of viruses and germs, knowing that even if they survive to middle age with their 'health' insurance fully paid up, they can soon anticipate the onset of heart disease or cancer? These diseases don't happen to animals in the wild whose bodies are no better designed than ours, in fact not nearly as good. Do they know something that we do not? The answer is no — to the contrary, we know something that they do not — we know how to take natural food and make it unnatural. We know how to take unnatural food and make it more unnatural, all the while making it delightful to eat although it strains our systems and pollutes our blood. We know how to arrange a diet to contain vast amounts of concentrated fat, cholesterol and protein, salt, sugar and condiments. And we know how to wash it all down with wine, coffee, tea and the milk of cows.

In short, we have elevated the practise of eating to an intensely pleasurable art form which unfortunately in the way it is commonly practised, overloads our vital organs, pollutes our blood and lymph, and diminishes our immune systems. Our cells get sick and we get sick.

The good news is that by changing to a diet of natural food the *milieu interieur* is quickly restored, and for most people well-being is theirs in just a few days.

CHAPTER THREE

Enzymes — The Secret Of Life

All forms of life on Earth are sustained by energy from the sun. The sun not only maintains a favorable warm environment and the energy to create weather, clouds and rain, it provides also the energy which is caught and stored in the green leaves of plants and in their fruits and seeds.

The complicated chemical processes involved in the growth of plants are possible only in the presence of enzymes, chemical catalysts without which no form of life — plant or animal — could exist.

When life first appeared on Earth there was little or no oxygen in the atmosphere, but eventually various bacteria evolved which could obtain energy from sunlight by photosynthesis, a process which results in the release of free oxygen previously contained in chemical compounds in the earth and atmosphere. With the increasing amount of available oxygen, higher forms of life began to evolve, leading eventually to the further evolution of plants and animals which of course are both aerobic forms of life (oxygen dependent).

The teeming myriads of micro-organisms that have for eons manufactured the Earth's topsoil and maintained its fertility, still form an essential link in the lives of both plants and animals because plants need them in soil as well as they need sun, air and rain — and animals in turn rely one way or another entirely on the plant kingdom to supply them with oxygen and nourishment.

The micro-organisms in their turn, break down dead vegetable and animal matter, and so the cycle continues...

All forms of life are inter-dependent, and none could exist without enzymes.

The following description of enzymes is taken from information provided by Dr Edward Howell of Fort Myers, Florida, who has made food enzymes a lifetime study, and is repeated from *The Health Revolution,* chapter 6.

Have you watched a jumbo-jet rise into the air, its wheels folding neatly out of sight as it speeds away to some distant land? Guided by electronic devices and computers, the pilot by radio, can speak, if he wishes, to either the local air traffic controller or to his home base, perhaps on the opposite side of the world. The traffic controller observes the aircraft's progress as a coded dot of light moving on a radar screen, and in the airplane itself the passengers can watch the latest movies. Powering the airplane and its 1,001 devices and computers are great jet engines burning vast quantities of carbon and hydrogen in the form of kerosene from large tanks in the wings.

The aircraft vanishes into the distance, leaving a white vapor trail high in the sky. You reflect on the wonders of civilization, the complexity of it all . . .

Powered also by carbon and hydrogen (from food), combining with the oxygen from the atmosphere, are the microscopic cells of the body, each one a thousand times more complex than any jumbo-jet. Reflect again. Imagine, as you read these words, the chemical and electrical processes going on inside your brain. Imagine the same processes, stepped up, in the minds and bodies of two tennis players contesting a hard match, or say a jazz saxophone player improvizing a hot solo — senses racing, fingers moving in a blur. Thoughts, actions and reactions — how can they occur so fast, billions of body cells so perfectly co-ordinated?

ENZYMES!

Every one of the countless processes within the body requires energy, released without the severe heat of fire, with exact precision, at a speed too fast to comprehend. Enzymes make this possible.

As school students all know, chemical reactions can be speeded up by the use of catalysts — chemicals which, without changing in form themselves, can influence other chemicals to combine and change at great speed. Because they remain unchanged, catalysts can be used over and over again. Enzymes act as catalysts in the body, enabling the release of energy and the operation of metabolic processes to occur at lightning speed.

Enzymes, however, have characteristics surpassing those of chemical catalysts and appear to hold the key to the mystery of life itself. They have been described as possessing properties intermediate between dead colloids and living cells, and to carry outside of the cell certain properties belonging to living matter. Unlike simple chemical catalysts which may last indefinitely, enzymes are gradually worn out as they accomplish their work, and must be constantly replenished.

Enzymes perform two separate but overlapping functions in the body:

1. The constant metabolism to do with tissue maintenance and general body functions.
2. The digestion of food.

Enzymes, which are protein-like substances, are produced in countless forms by the body, and countless thousands of combinations or systems. Each enzyme exists for a specific purpose and there is not one body process — thought, digestion, movement or growth — that can occur without enzyme activity. Life, animal or vegetable, cannot exist without enzymes. For all intents and purposes, life and enzyme activity are one and the same. Enzyme levels in the body can be measured, and it is a fact that even though vitamins and mineral levels remain fairly constant throughout life, enzyme levels do not; they are highest in young adulthood and decline with age. Enzyme levels rise in acute illness, if the body has the resources, but are always low in chronic disease.

Dr. Edward Howell, in his book *The Status of Food Enzymes in Digestion and Metabolism,** says: "The fact that the enzyme content of organisms is depleted with increasing old age is forcibly presented when fluids or tissues are examined at different ages. After full mature growth has been attained there is a slow and gradual decrease in the enzyme content of organisms. When the enzyme content becomes so low that metabolism cannot proceed at a proper level, death overtakes the organism". This decline in enzyme production is explainable by the silting up and degeneration of the body cells which, it appears, is the cause of the problem and not a result of it.

Enzyme activity requires the presence of moisture, and varies with temperature and the degree of acidity present. Some enzymes function in an acid environment, others prefer neutral conditions, and some alkaline. Maximum activity occurs at different temperatures depending on the acid/alkaline balance, and at different degrees of acidity depending on the temperature. In the body, enzymes function more rapidly and more effort can be produced at temperatures above normal. Enzyme activity reaches a maximum at fever temperatures which accompany acute infection, thus accomplishing maximum action by the body's defensive mechanisms.

In 1921, Professor Eugene Du Bois described in the Journal of the American Medical Association that a rise in temperature from the normal 37 °C (98.6 °F) to 41°C (105 °F) produced a 50% increase in the metabolism of the human body. In 1926, Dr. S. Wright in his *Applied Physiology* stated that for every rise of one degree Fahrenheit, the basal metabolism increases by

*Dr Howell's books *The Status of Food Enzymes in Digestion and Metabolism,* 1946, (reprinted as *Food Enzymes for Health and Longevity,* 1980) and *Enzyme Nutrition,* 1983, are essential reading for all students of nutrition. Without the information provided by Dr Howell, the science of nutrition cannot proceed beyond 'first base'.

seven per cent.

The normal human body temperature ranges from 36 °C (97 °F) at between 2 and 5 a.m. when the metabolism is slowest, to 37.2 °C (99 °F) at between 2 and 5 p.m. when the metabolism is greatest.

These facts, in addition to explaining the function of fever, also explain why it is necessary for athletes to "warm-up" before competition and why drowning people survive longer in cold water.

Above 42 °C (107 °F) enzymes eventually become impaired and if enzymes in raw food are heated to 48° (118 °F) for more than half an hour they are destroyed. It should be noted that the destructive effects of heat are most pronounced when moisture is present. Dry heat is not destructive to enzymes until temperatures above 150 °C (302 °F) and at lower temperatures than this extracted enzymes in powder form suffer no damage.

Cold blooded organisms such as insects or reptiles, have body temperatures which vary with the temperature of their surroundings and are sluggish or inactive in cold weather, becoming active in the summer or when able to bask in the sun. In experiments, the metabolism of insects can be speeded enormously by increasing the temperature, but at the same time this greatly shortens their lifespan. Slow moving creatures such as tortoises are capable of living to a great age, and so too are elephants, also slow moving. Elephants have an average body temperature of 35.5 °C (96 °F), whereas fast moving creatures such as small birds have body temperatures of 42 °C (108 °F) and are short lived.

Seeds contain enzymes which are inhibited until exposed to conditions of moisture and temperature favorable to germination. Thus in temperate climates new growth commences in the spring, and maximum growth occurs in the summer. In damp tropical climates lush growth occurs all year round.

The enzyme potential of seeds is inhibited by specific inhibiting agents in the seed which ensure the seed remains inert and apparently lifeless, perhaps for years, until conditions favorable to germination are encountered. Cooked food keeps well because its natural enzymes which would otherwise decompose it, have been destroyed, and it will only decompose when live enzymes are introduced by various microbes in the air. Because enzymes are inhibited by cold, refrigerated food keeps well and frozen food will keep indefinitely. Similarly, dehydrated food will keep indefinitely because enzymes cannot function without moisture. Canned food also keeps indefinitely because its enzymes have been destroyed by heat and the food sealed in the can from further enzyme contact. Preservatives work by inhibiting enzymes and this is why preserved foods are difficult to digest.

All living organic matter, animal or vegetable, lives only because of enzyme activity, and upon death it is decomposed and returned to the earth by enzyme activity.

The digestion and assimilation of food requires that the food be broken down into constituents which can be absorbed and utilized by the body. Protein must be broken down into usable amino-acids, starch into sugar, and fats split into simple components. Minerals and vitamins must be extracted and either put to immediate use or stored away. All of these actions are accomplished by about a dozen different digestive enzymes acting separately and together. Some of these enzymes exist already in the food if it is uncooked, but the majority are provided in the digestive juices made in the body and secreted into the stomach and intestines. The pancreas provides some of these but most are provided by the cells of the intestinal villi.

Because cooked food can be digested with apparent ease by most people, it is maintained by some authorities that cooking is relatively harmless to food, depleting only a little from its nourishment. It is also maintained that the destruction of food enzymes by cooking means nothing because the enzymes are supposedly destroyed anyhow in the acid medium of the stomach before the food reaches the intestine. This argument is wrong, it has been shown over and over again that although some of them are destroyed in the stomach, exogenous enzymes (i.e. from outside the body) contained in raw food play an important part not only in assisting the digestive processes, thus relieving the pancreas of extra work, but in addition, are absorbed into the lymph and blood stream to supplement enzyme production within the body.

Dr. Howell describes how the digestive enzymes secreted by humans eating cooked foods, are much stronger than those secreted by animals eating raw food, and how the human pancreas is hypertrophied due to overwork. He says: "A separate and distinct organ, the food enzyme stomach, is widespread in Nature. It was evolved specifically to pre-digest food by food enzymes before the body's digestive enzymes come into contact with the food. I have also documented that three outstanding, authoritative texts, *Gray's Anatomy*, *Cunningham's Anatomy* and *Howell's Physiology* have recorded that the human stomach consists essentially of two parts — the upper section and the lower section, with different physiological duties. The upper part of the human stomach performs the same function as the food-enzyme stomach of animals, which is the pre-digestion of food by food enzymes."

The enzyme content of natural food is proportional to the amount of energy (calories) contained. Raw vegetables do not contain a great quantity of enzymes and so salads do little to compensate for the destruction of enzymes in cooked food. Fruit is high in enzyme content. Fruit will ripen rapidly then decompose rapidly in hot weather, while vegetables may only wilt and shrivel. Animal protein foods, meat, fat and dairy products when raw contain valuable enzymes.

Whereas the enzymes of the body's digestive juices or of manufactured enzyme supplements are much stronger than enzymes in raw food, the consumption of raw food stimulates the secretion of weaker hydrochloric acid into the stomach so that exogenous enzymes in the food can perform longer and with greater effect before being neutralized.

Dr. Howell describes experiments which show that it is possible for unsplit, complex substances such as bacteria, yeast cells, proteins and fats to be absorbed into the bloodstream and lymph. Such substances in the body fluids are foreign and therefore antigenic, provoking allergic responses and leucocytosis, the increase in the blood's white cells. The experiments showed that enzymes in the blood serum, if adequate, complete the digestion of these substances. It was shown too, that when enzyme levels were low and symptoms of allergy were present, these symptoms subsided and enzyme levels returned to normal after large doses of pancreatic enzymes were administered orally to the patient.

It is argued that cereal foods must be cooked for them to be digested, and this is true for the following reasons: firstly, heat is needed to burst the cellulose envelope surrounding the starch in the cereal so that the digestive juices can get access to the starch, and secondly, the heat not only destroys the natural enzymes but also the enzyme inhibitors which would otherwise prevent the pancreatic enzymes working. In this way cereals can be digested, but more so than with any other cooked food, so many extra digestive enzymes are required that the pancreas is overworked.

Nuts, considered generally as health food, are seeds and contain enzyme inhibitors which must be neutralized by heat before they can be properly digested. The best way of obtaining nourishment from seeds and nuts is by germinating them and consuming them raw.

The regular consumption of cooked food results in the enlargement of the pancreas, and hypertrophy of this organ is the most pronounced in people who consume large amounts of cooked grains (including rice). By comparison, as a percentage of total body weight the human pancreas is over twice the size of the pancreas of herbivorous animals, the only explanation being that humans consume cooked food. Experiments at the University of Minnesota showed that when rats were put on a diet containing 80% heat treated carbohydrate carefully constructed to contain all nutrients and vitamins, the pancreas and sub-maxillary glands increased in weight 20-30% in a period of 155 days.

Thus, notwithstanding the fact that cereals of one kind or another constitute the basis of the diets of most humans, this form of food cannot contribute to optimal nutrition. What constitutes optimal nutrition is discussed in later chapters.

Accompanying the hypertrophy of the pancreas brought about in the digestion of cooked food are changes in the gonads, adrenals, pituitary and other ductless glands. A study of people killed accidentally showed that all of those over fifty had a defective pituitary gland, which is the master gland of the body.

To say that enlargement of the pancreas demonstrates the capability of the body to adapt, is an argument valid only in the short term. Our object is health and longevity. It was proposed by a health professional in a lecture I heard recently, that manufactured dog food, scientifically prepared to contain a perfect balance of nutrients, was capable of providing perfect nutrition for humans too. Why not? Laboratory animals fed similar scientifically prepared food appear to maintain good health. Such observations however, are not valid because the test animals are always young ones whose lives are terminated before degeneration is evident. In experiments where rats have been kept several years on manufactured food only, the animals have been observed after only two years to develop a variety of pathological conditions commonly suffered by aged humans, including blindness in half of them, followed by death soon afterwards.

To conclude with some further remarks from Dr. Howell: "At first thought it might be presumed that hypertrophy of the pancreas is a desirable accommodation. But there is always the tendency for the hypertrophy of excessive function to proceed to the atrophy of exhaustion. An atrophy of the pancreas occurs in many terminal wasting diseases".

Dr. Howell's whole argument is that if throughout life the enzyme production within the body is overstrained, in the later years it is inevitable that enzyme levels will diminish sooner than they should, thus accelerating degeneration and old age. Referring to an experiment at Cornell University in which it was shown that the lifespan of rats could be almost doubled by dietary manipulation, Dr. Howell said. "After reviewing this work, I cannot see how it is possible to escape the conclusion that when the enzyme reserve (I use this phrase interchangeably with the term vitality) is drawn at a more rapid rate it will be exhausted sooner and consequently life will end earlier".

The foregoing information about enzymes gives, of course, only an inkling of the vital part they play in the metabolism of all living things, and of how the metabolism of all animal organisms is totally dependent in the first place on the enzyme metabolism of the plants which provide their sustenance. Without some comprehension of these things the study of nutrition cannot properly proceed, and conclusions drawn will to a great extent, be erroneous.

CHAPTER FOUR

Human Nutrition

Towards the end of World War II when the Americans invaded the Philippines and recaptured them from the Japanese, a lone Japanese soldier ran off into the jungle there and hid, firmly believing that sooner or later the tide of battle would turn again and Japan would in the end be victorious. He therefore decided to wait things out in the jungle. He waited 25 years, all the while avoiding human contact, and then one day emerged from the jungle and surrendered.

Returned to Japan and medically examined, the soldier amazed everybody — he looked so young compared to other middle-aged Japanese men. His teeth were perfect and his eyesight too. He displayed none of the usual signs of degenerative disease considered normal in civilization. And yet his life had not been easy. The only possible explanation for his physical preservation was that his diet for 25 years had been fruit, berries and various plants eaten raw — a diet similar to that of other wild primates and that of early humans before the discovery of fire . . .

The natural diet of man

Life of all kinds is most prolific in tropical regions both on land and sea, and this is not to be wondered at because it is in warm and moist conditions that enzymes work most efficiently. In such a warm, moist environment it is thought that life first appeared on Earth, and it is generally accepted that it was in the tropics that the early primates evolved from lower forms of life, to be followed by the evolution of the apes and then by the first humans.

In the plant kingdom, fruit trees were late arrivals on the evolutionary scene and it is highly probable that both fruit bearing trees and the primates evolved concurrently, which accounts for the development in the primates of stereoscopic color vision, grasping hands, specialized teeth and jaw structure, appetite for sweet tasting food, medium length digestive tract, and so on. In their symbionic relationship, the fruit trees provided the primates with food and the primates unknowingly spread the fruit seeds wherever they ate or defecated, so ensuring the continued survival of the trees.

The study of comparative anatomy and the different natural diets of animals in the wild indicates strongly that the natural diet of early humans consisted predominantly of sweet fruits, and that even though millions of years have passed, the anatomy and digestive apparatus of humans has not changed and is therefore still best suited to fruit as the most suitable food. That this opinion is not just idle speculation can be quickly proven by any sick person who can break the addiction to our modern taste-stimulating foods and go on a diet of good quality fruit for just a few days. Of course the human digestive system is quite capable of handling foods of animal origin, including animal fats, but in only very limited amounts can it do so without strain, even when the foods are eaten raw as intended by Nature.

Thus it can be surmised that the ideal diet for man is one mainly of sweet fruits supplemented by various berries, green nuts, shoots and occasionally small amounts of foods of animal origin, all eaten raw. This is the sort of food eaten by man's closest relatives in Nature, the orang-outang and chimpanzee, both of which have an anatomy and digestive system almost identical to man's. Neither of these animals in the wild displays tooth decay or any of the other diseases common to humans but soon do so if kept in captivity and fed cooked and processed food.

If this surmise is correct, and if indeed humans can live in better health and for a longer time on such a natural diet, why ever did they change?

Civilization and civilized disease

There is not a race of people anywhere today who, as a general rule, eat uncooked natural food; the majority of the world's populations base their diets on cooked grains of some kind or other, and the rest base theirs on cooked animal products supplemented by grain, dairy products and vegetables, all cooked. Fruit is looked upon more as a mere accessory to the various traditional diets rather than a sustaining food. How and why did this change come about?

Early man lived in small groups, and before the use of fire, ate his food raw like all the other creatures on Earth have done since life first began, their senses of sight, smell and taste indicating to them the foods most suitable to their systems. Population numbers were restricted by the amount of food available growing wild, but eventually with the discovery of fire it was found that various foods consumed by other animals but which were distasteful to the human palate, could be made more edible by cooking, and more tasteful by artificially flavoring them with herbs and salt.

By the use of these new sources of food, greater populations could be supported, not only in areas already occupied, but in territory where food naturally suited for humans was not available. As population pressures forced surplus people to move into less hospitable territory outside the tropics, they of necessity became reliant on a different diet, and on fire and primitive clothing for warmth.

Greater challenges in a less benevolent environment led to continued brain development, and so it was in the temperate climatic zones of the world that technology commenced, leading to the advent of farming and the development of cereal crops from wild grasses. Continued competition for territory made warfare inevitable and this led again to greater technological development and so on. From all these changes a new breed of man emerged — one who had become 'civilized' and had left his natural environment forever.

Next to the discovery of fire, the development of grain crops was the greatest factor leading to the human population explosion of today. Grain could be produced easily, and being storable, provided food for all seasons. More and more forest land was destroyed to grow crops and to make pasture to raise cattle, and according to their circumstances some populations came to base their diets on meat and dairy products and others based theirs on rice or wheat or other sorts of grain.

None of these diets provide ideal nutrition, and as civilization 'progresses' and food becomes more and more preserved, processed, cooked, and generally less and less natural, so humans everywhere display more signs of disease earlier and earlier in life. Even primitive races have always had their medicine men to protect their people from evil spirits and disease, but in civilization the superstition of medicine has got out of hand; 'scientific medicine' has become a powerful industry consuming a vast amount of the national economy. But while the wild animals remain sleek and healthy without medicine, humans spend more and more money on 'health care' and all the while just get sicker and sicker. We have now reached the stage where — apart from accidents — degenerative diseases of one kind or another account almost entirely for all deaths in the modern countries, three out of four for a start being due to heart disease and cancer. As will be described later, not only are heart disease and cancer caused primarily by incorrect nutrition, but so too are the other 'diseases of civilization'.

The only solution to our health problems then is to abandon our reliance on modern medicine, which for all its science still flounders in ignorance, and to address the underlying basic cause of the problems, which is the subtle addiction to foods that stimulate but improperly nourish.

What is correct nourishment?

To assess the correctness of a diet we must first understand the purpose to which the body puts the components supplied in food.

The body is a very complicated machine which like any other must be kept in good repair and supplied with fuel to provide the energy to keep it going. And like other machines which are of high quality and good design, the body requires little expenditure on repairs and maintenance, most of its needs being in the form of fuel. And if the fuel supplied is pure and 'clean-burning' the body will not clog up with residues and will run smoothly and efficiently for a very long time. The advantage the body has over ordinary machines is that it is entirely self-regulating, and given the right materials it can repair itself without any outside help whatever. Its big disadvantage is that once it grinds to a halt you cannot start it ever again . . .

Food provides the body with the following substances:

1. ***Materials for growth and repair.*** These are amino acids and minerals of different kinds which may be obtained from vegetable sources or by the breaking down of existing protein from animal sources. Existing protein must be broken down by digestion into its amino acid components which are then used to construct any new protein needed by the body. As the body is capable of recycling a lot of the materials from worn out cells etc., only very little protein and minerals need be contained in the diet. Scientific studies have shown that healthy adults can maintain normal metabolism and activity on a diet containing as little as 3% protein as a percentage of total calories (about 20 grams per day).
2. ***Materials for energy production (fuel).*** These can be in the form of carbohydrates, fat and protein. Carbohydrates are the

best sources of energy because they metabolise in the body most efficiently to provide energy, producing as byproducts only carbon dioxide and water, both of which are perfectly harmless substances easily expelled from the body. The water formed is pure, and useful for other body functions.

When the diet contains more than the minimum of protein or fat needed by the body, the excess is used for energy production, but as protein and fat are not 'clean-burning' fuels, toxic byproducts are produced in the form of ammonia and uric acid from the protein, and ketones from the fats; so not only is an extra load placed on the body in converting the protein and fat into energy, but then further work must be done to eliminate their toxic byproducts (see "Water", end of chapter).

This is why diets high in protein and fat cause degeneration of the vital organs, particularly the kidneys.

A diet of completely natural vegetarian food may contain as little as 3% protein and 3% fat which are adequate amounts for a fully-grown adult, the remaining 94% being in the form of carbohydrate. Such a diet is ideal for the human system because all the body's needs are met with little formation of harmful substances of any kind.

3. ***Vitamins and minerals.*** These are used by the body to perform the various complex processes of food digestion and general metabolism. The body manufactures all the enzymes it needs from protein and various minerals, and these work in conjunction with the vitamins which are sometimes referred to as co-enzymes.
4. ***Dietary fiber.*** All vegetable substances, unrefined, contain fiber which is formed mainly of cellulose and is only partially digestible. Fiber gives bulk to the food substances and allows the digestive tract to keep the digesting food moving, thus allowing an easy transit through the body and freeing the body of constipation. Animal substances — meat, fish, dairy products and fat — contain no fiber at all and nor do refined and processed

carbohydrates such as white flour and sugar. This is why diets based on these foods invariably cause constipation together with their other harmful effects.

That completes the list of minimum requirements to be furnished from the diet as most nutritionists would agree, although they may dispute the low percentages given for protein and fat. But is the list really complete?

Food enzymes

Proteins, carbohydrates, fats, minerals and vitamins — is that all the body requires? Dr Edward Howell asked himself that question as a practising doctor in 1932. Animal experiments had indicated that proteins, carbohydrates, fats, minerals and vitamins provided the complete spectrum needed for human nutrition, but there were many researchers who claimed that natural raw food was better for you — it contained a vital factor, a vital force of some kind. Dr Howell raised the question again, what about enzymes?

Speaking today Dr Howell says: "I thought I should investigate the subject of enzymes in food and I figured that two years reading all the research data would be sufficient time." — pause — "That was fifty-five years ago, and I'm still at it!" The reason Dr Howell could not complete his project in two years was that when he started combing all the research material for information he could find nothing. Nobody had ever before made a study of food enzymes, so he had to start out on his own. Dr Howell remained in medical practise until 1970, spending three days a week tending his patients and the rest of the time in food enzyme research. Since 1970 his research has been full time.

Dr Howell's research findings (see books referred to in chapter 3) fill a huge gap in the traditional ideas on nutrition and make possible, for the first time, a full comprehension of the subject.

As explained briefly in chapter 3, enzymes in fresh raw food exist not only for metabolic life processes while the food plant (or animal) is alive, but also to break down its tissues so that they can return to the earth again after death. This process of decomposition is called autolysis and is universal in Nature. . . 'From dust thou art and to dust thou shall return' (per action of enzymes).

When fresh, raw food is eaten, the process of autolysis, instead of proceeding on the floor of the jungle, proceeds instead in the upper (cardiac) part of the human stomach (some animals have a separate stomach for this purpose) and proceeds at an accelerated rate because the conditions of moisture and temperature in the stomach are ideally suited for the action of the autolytic enzymes contained in the food itself. This decomposition of food proceeds for periods up to one hour depending on the kind of food. Thus a substantial degree of pre-digestion is accomplished in the cardiac section before the food begins to mix with the acidic protein-splitting gastric juices in the lower (pyloric) section of the stomach where the food enzymes to a greater or lesser extent become inactivated. Whatever the nature of the raw food — protein, carbohydrate or fat — the required autolytic enzymes — protease, amylase or lipase — are already present in the food itself to commence the predigestive process. The only predigestive enzyme produced by the body is the starch-splitting enzyme ptyalin (amylase) which appears in the saliva when starchy foods are eaten, and which initiates the breakdown of starch into sugar. Thus the digestion of starch commences in the mouth, with the ptyalin continuing its action in the stomach for a considerable time until inactivated by the acidic gastric juices there, whose concentration varies with the amount of protein to be digested. This facility enables the digestive system to handle fruits which are not quite ripe, in which case their carbohydrates are as yet only partially converted to fruit sugar. Unripe fruit is sour to taste and cannot be swallowed until thoroughly chewed, whereupon the action of the ptyalin sweetens the chewed morsel, signalling the go-ahead to swallow. Ptyalin will work on cooked starchy carbohydrate but only if the food is dry and then thoroughly chewed. Wet or greasy flavoured starch fools the taste receptors and so the starch, enzymeless, proceeds to the stomach (as does cooked fat) and sits there for several hours, giving rise to the feeling of fullness and indigestion. Thus complex carbohydrates (starch foods) may be digested quickly (to account for the high glycemic rating of bread referred to in chapter 1), or slowly if their digestive process is delayed in the absence of ptyalin.

The text-books on nutrition don't mention these interesting events because the people who write the text-books don't know about them. However, the digestive events which occur in the lower stomach, the duodenum, intestine and bowel are generally well understood, involving as they do the activity of digestive enzymes produced within the body itself. But nobody except Dr Howell has stopped to query why the human pancreas is up to three times bigger than it should be when compared size for size with those of all other animals. It has been queried often enough, however, why flesh eating animals are not troubled by cholesterol, and why primitive Eskimos, who eat their meat and fat raw, have low cholesterol levels and are untroubled by blood fats. The answer to these queries lies in the autolytic breakdown of raw food in the stomach by the enzymes contained in the food itself. When these enzymes are present all is well, but when they are destroyed by cooking and completely missing, the pancreas has to work overtime to produce extra enzymes in an endeavour to accomplish the stage of digestion that has been entirely missed.

The importance of enzymes in food is not only that a load is taken off the pancreas, but possibly more important, the food is more completely broken down before assimilation from the intestine, so reducing the workload on the liver and at the same time permitting more efficient metabolic processes throughout the entire body. The observations of researchers, Doctors Harvarth, Edward Howell, Maynard Murray, Peter Heinbecker,

J. M. Rabinowitch, J. A. Urquhart and others, described in the paper, 'Lipase versus Cholesterol' (1983) by Dr Howell, demonstrate this fact.

When improperly digested (i.e. not properly broken down) food substances enter the bloodstream they are antigenic to the body and provoke attack by the white cells of the immune system which cells use their own digestive enzymes to destroy the particles. If the white cells fail to accomplish their job properly the remaining food particles, usually in the form of protein molecules, cause reactions of various kinds known as allergy reaction.

The value of enzymes in raw fruit and vegetables is well known, but just as important are the enzymes in foods of animal origin. Animal protein, raw, contains the proteolytic enzyme cathepsin, and animal fat, raw, contains adipose lipase. All these food enzymes work to predigest their particular food component in the upper (cardiac) section of the stomach before being inactivated by the gastric acid during the mixing action in the lower stomach, which acid will be less concentrated anyhow because of the predigestion already accomplished. The research shows that the resultant more thorough breakdown of these foods in the intestine enables the body to more efficiently metabolize the protein, fat and cholesterol, thereby reducing the tendency to atherosclerosis and other problems.

It is preferable that food should be eaten at about body temperature; if food is eaten cold or hot, digestive action cannot proceed until the food has warmed or cooled to the temperature at which enzymes work.

If raw food is allowed to 'ripen' before eating, such as when meat is hung for several days, it becomes actually partially pre-digested by its own enzymes. This breakdown of the food substances referred to here as 'pre-digestion' is in fact merely the process of autolysis by which all living things are decomposed so they can return to the earth and become part of it again. In 1935, Dr Urquhart, in the *Canadian Medical Association Journal,* described how Eskimos did not cut up caribou meat until the animal had been dead for a few days. Similarly, freshly caught fish were buried to be later eaten uncooked in a partly decomposed state. The Eskimos gained a health benefit from this practise, said Dr Urquhart who described from his own experience how hard-working sled dogs could maintain top condition on such food whereas on a diet of fresh fish they weakened and lost weight after two weeks.

Further evidence that natural enzymes in uncooked food play a significant part in the digestive process is the fact that herbivorous animals although requiring large quantities of digestive enzymes, have none in their saliva and have a pancreas of less than half the size compared with their body weight, than humans, who eat mainly cooked food. This shows that the digestive enzymes required by the animals must be furnished mainly in their food.

Allowing for differences in anatomy and so on, that this comparison is valid is indicated by the fact that hypertrophy of the pancreas of animals occurs when their diet is changed to heat denatured, enzyme-deficient food. As already mentioned, experiments by Dr Jackson, Department of Anatomy, University of Minnesota, showed that on such a diet, otherwise properly balanced, in a period of 155 days the pancreas and submaxillary glands of rats increased in weight by 20-30%, while the pituitary and suprarenals decreased in weight.

Accompanying the enlargement of the pancreas brought about in the digestion of cooked food are changes in the gonads, adrenals, pituitary and other ductless glands. A study of people killed accidentally showed that all those over fifty had a defective pituitary gland, the master gland of the body.

Another report by Dr Arnold Renshaw of England in *The Annals of Rheumatic Disease* (1947), based on thousands of autopsy observations, noted that atrophy of the small intestine was a constant finding.

The importance of pre-digestion by food enzymes in the cardiac section of the stomach cannot be over-estimated. As Dr Howell points out, the body's health and endurance is dependent entirely on efficient metabolism, which in turn is entirely dependent on the action of enzymes, and its youthfulness and vitality is directly proportional to the levels of enzymes contained in its tissues and blood. To repeat, when enzymeless cooked food is consumed, a most important digestive function is entirely eliminated, throwing extra strain on the digestive system and consuming part of the body's vital enzyme reserves. That the body can cope there is no doubt, but the strain is indicated by the hypertrophy of the pancreas, the enlargement of the liver, and changes in other vital organs, leading to diminished vitality and premature old-age.

Salt

Salt is mentioned here because some people think that, in moderation, it is harmless and in fact even a form of nutrient providing the body with sodium. Even though Pritikin advised against salt, mainly for the reason it can cause edema from which stem "a host of circulatory problems", he still permitted up to four grams (a half teaspoon) per day.

Salt, in the form of common salt or sea salt (sodium chloride) is a poison. It inhibits enzyme activity in or out of the body, and this is why it performs so well as a preservative and why preserved food causes digestive complications. In addition, its capacity to draw water to itself makes it a powerful irritant, destroying fragile cells in the mouth and along the digestive tract as well as causing edema within the body tissues. To Dr Max Gerson (see chapter 8), salt was the most offensive article of diet used by humans.

How balanced is the traditional 'balanced' diet?

The conventional concept of good nutrition is that one should eat a balanced diet. By this is meant the diet, in order to provide the body with all its needs, should contain approximately equal proportions of the main food groups: animal protein foods (meat, fish, poultry and eggs), dairy products (milk and cheese), grain products (cereals, bread, pasta etc.), and vegetables and fruit.

This concept is based on assumptions which are gravely false, and accordingly is the main reason underlying the diseases of civilization.

The false assumptions are:

1. That animal protein is essential and that vegetable protein is inferior.
2. That protein should be copiously supplied.
3. That animal protein is necessary to provide vitamin B_{12}.
4. That the diet should contain a moderate amount of fat.
5. That grain products are desirable foods.
6. That dairy products are necessary to provide calcium.
7. That dairy products are wholesome.
8. That pasteurization is desirable.
9. That cooking does little to deplete the value of food.

Comments

- The most powerful animals in the world such as elephants and oxen derive all their protein from completely vegetarian sources. All animal proteins, even grubs in apples, come from amino acids derived from vegetable sources. Humans can easily derive all the protein they need from either vegetables or fruit, without the intake of nuts or grains.
- As already mentioned, human adults need only 3% to 4% of their total dietary calories as protein, and this amount is available from a fruitarian diet or a vegetarian diet, without supplementation by cereals or nuts. Mothers' breast milk contains only 6% protein, and this provides for the most rapid rate of growth a human ever attains, when a baby can double its birth weight in six months or less. The problem when arranging a proper diet is not in getting enough protein but

in keeping protein down to safe levels. Even the Pritikin regression diet, which contains only a mere trace of animal protein, contains excessive amounts of protein by virtue of the fact the diet is based on the intake of grain products. The grain products are included in the Pritikin diet to provide desirable levels of complex carbohydrate, but besides the carbohydrates in grains being in the undesirable form of starch, the protein level in grains can be as high as 12%, sufficient to cause metabolic upsets in the body. (More of this later.)

- Apart from the mischief caused by the toxic byproducts of protein metabolism, protein digestion results in severe inroads of the body's energy reserves largely because of the amount of hydrochloric acid required, as described in Professor Arthur C. Guyton's *Textbook of Medical Physiology:* "The laws of energy conservation require energy expenditure any time the concentration of a specific ion is changed from low concentration to high concentration. Consequently, concentrating the hydrogen ion from the normal pH of body fluids at 7.4 to a pH of less than 1.0 requires the expenditure of large quantities of energy by the parietal cells. This fact is mentioned to emphasize the necessity for tremendous energy expenditure by essentially all glandular cells of the body."
- It has been shown that vitamin B_{12} need not be present in the human diet as it can be synthesized by bacteria in the digestive tract. There are many absolute vegetarians (vegans) who maintain perfect health without ever touching animal food of any kind. Dr Richard Bargen, in his book *The Vegetarian's Self-Defense Manual* (1979) described his exhaustive research on this subject and summed up by saying, "After a careful review of all the literature often quoted as demonstrating 'pure' vegetarians often suffer from a vitamin B_{12} deficiency because of inadequate dietary intake, not one solitary case was found wherein a vegan consuming an adequate purely plant food diet suffered any ill health due to vitamin B_{12} deficiency or any other

deficiency. This finding contradicts the statements made in virtually every textbook of medicine and nutrition I've ever come across."

- The typical 'balanced' diet contains up to 45% of its calories in fat, which is a dangerous amount. Medical authorities recommend 30% which is still a dangerous amount.

  The diet of wild primates contains about 4% fat and studies of primitive New Guinea natives show them to maintain vigorous health on a diet containing only 4% fat. All vegetables and fruit contain small amounts of fat, amounts which are more than adequate for humans. There is no need to 'include' fats in the diet, any more than there is to 'include' protein in the diet, because all ordinary foodstuffs contain more than enough of both.

  It is commonly believed that vegetable fats should be used in the diet in place of animal fats because vegetable fats are unsaturated and are free of cholesterol. It is true that animal fats should be avoided but it is absolutely unnecessary and just as dangerous to use extracted vegetable oils which have been shown to just as adversely affect the viscosity of the blood as other fats and indeed have been shown to increase the risk of cancer.
- The faults of grains are many. (See chapter 10.)
- Humans are the only creatures on Earth that drink milk after they have been weaned and then it is the milk of other animals they use. Humans are the only animals that commonly suffer tooth decay and osteoporosis. Oxen and other powerful herbivorous animals, like all the other vegetarian creatures, get adequate amounts of calcium for strong bones and teeth from grass and other vegetable matter. Vegetarian people do not suffer osteoporosis, it is the big protein eater that does because the body draws calcium from the bones to try and neutralize the acid formed in the system by the metabolism of protein. It is a fallacy that taking milk or calcium tablets can help

someone with osteoporosis; what they need is less protein and more exercise. Carnivorous animals have a system designed to more efficiently dispose of the waste products of protein metabolism, but it is significant that they never prey on each other, only on herbivorous creatures.

- Dairy products are not desirable foodstuffs for humans of any age, but if used they are far better unpasteurized. There are about 35 different enzymes in milk, all of which are destroyed by pasteurization. Milk and especially cheese are high in fat and contain cholesterol, and patients on milk diets for stomach ulcers rapidly develop atherosclerosis of the arteries. Of all foods, cow's milk is responsible for the highest rate of allergy reactions in humans and has been found responsible for causing all kinds of psychiatric disorders. Young children reared on a vegetarian diet without milk of any kind maintain normal rates of growth and at the same time remain mucous free and do not have the problem of bed wetting which is another complaint found to be associated with milk drinking.

• The Effect of Cooking and the Value of Raw Food

There is no doubt that the cooking of food is an unnatural process invented by man comparatively recently in his evolutionary development. Although cooking may render certain foods, such as cereals, more readily assimilable to human digestion, and render some foods more palatable, generally it is a destructive process which seriously depletes the nutritive value of food.

It has been explained that animal life is totally dependent on the plant kingdom for oxygen and food. Plants convert inorganic chemicals from the earth, air and water into organic plant forms from which animals can derive nourishment. Inorganic substances cannot nourish animals. When fresh food is cooked it is to a greater or lesser extent converted back to inorganic compounds again and the longer and hotter the cookery process the less the nourishment and the greater the toxicity the food will provide.

Dr Herbert Shelton, referred to earlier, in his book *Superior Nutrition,* said: "Cooking destroys in part, if not wholly, the oxidizable factors of foods. This simply means that cooking 'burns' those portions of foods that the body ordinarily oxidizes. Once these substances have been oxidized, they cannot again be oxidized in the body, hence they are useless as food. Heat, by speeding up oxidization, turns food into ashes before it is eaten. For example, certain of the amino acids, lysine and glutamine are destroyed by the cooking process. The losses that are produced by cooking may not result in serious trouble until later in life and all of their effects do not show up for two or three generations."

Consider the following points:

1. When the nutritive value of food is decreased, more food must be eaten to achieve satisfaction of the appetite, and because the culinary art of cooking is designed to artificially stimulate the appetite, over-eating naturally follows.
2. All foods, particularly if cooked, to a greater or lesser extent introduce toxic substances into the body, which must be eliminated. Some toxins come directly from the food when digested and others are formed as byproducts of body metabolism. The more food eaten, the more toxins are produced, and the faster will be the degeneration of the body's vital organs.
3. Natural foods contain generous quantities of micronutrients — vitamins, minerals and enzymes — all of which are damaged in varying degrees by cooking. To metabolize cooked food, the body needs more micronutrients, not less, so that the consumer is put in a "Catch 22" situation, needing more but receiving less.
4. Apart from wear and tear on the vital organs, toxins and mineral wastes above the capacity of the body to eliminate, gradually accumulate in the arteries and other body tissues. This process is greatest when cooked food is eaten, and least with raw food.
5. Natural enzymes in fresh food are destroyed at temperatures above 48°C (118°F). While some authorities argue that this does

not matter because enzymes are destroyed anyhow by the acid in the stomach, there is much evidence to prove that not only do food enzymes achieve a significant degree of pre-digestion of food in the upper part of the stomach before being neutralized by stomach acid, but also sufficient enzymes survive to reach the intestine and are absorbed for use in the body.

6. When food or drink is heated above about 180°F a further damaging effect occurs which increases in severity with the degree of heat. When the cooled food is eaten, the body suffers a pathological challenge which is indicated by a sudden increase in the white cells in the blood, known as leucocytosis. Some highly processed meats for instance, may cause a white cell increase of 300%.

Although the reasons were not understood, the harmful effects of cooked food have long been known. In 1829, Vincent Priessnitz of Silesia described the 'inflamed and brittle' flesh of a pig which had been fed on cooked food all its life and compared it with the 'firm and healthy' flesh of pigs fed on raw food. A diet of raw fruit and vegetables formed the basis of treatment at Louis Kuhne's celebrated clinic in Leipzig, Germany, one hundred years ago, and has ever since been the basis of treatment in the many other famed sanatoriums of the world.

As already mentioned, the destruction of enzymes is not the only harm caused by heating food. Japanese experiments with baby mice showed that when fed milk which had previously been heated, the mice did not survive. Using milk previously heated to 80°C (176°F) for half an hour, mice survived only three weeks. The higher the temperature to which the milk was heated the shorter was the survival time — 120°C (248°F) caused death in one week, and 140°C (284°F) caused death in three to five days. The famous Pottenger experiment throws further light on this subject in view of the fact that raw meat was included in the cat's diet.

A medical paper, *The Effect of Heat Processed Foods and*

Metabolized Vitamin D Milk on the Dentofacial Structures of Experimental Animals by Dr Francis Pottenger (1946) described tests on cats where one group was fed raw milk, another group pasteurized milk, and a third group evaporated milk and condensed milk. The experiment was continued for four generations of cats.

All generations on the raw milk group thrived. The other two groups deteriorated from the start. They suffered a lowered condition and the second generation was depleted by stillbirth, miscarriage, spontaneous abortion, or resorption in the uterus. The survivors had many defects which included eczema, calcification of tissues, anatomical defects, neuroses and abnormalities in neuromuscular co-ordination. Anatomical differences between the sexes became less apparent and homosexuality appeared.

The third generation was greatly depleted and there was no fourth generation at all; there was not even an attempt at reproduction by the third generation.

The most significant fact revealed by this experiment, apart from the lethal effects on the experimental cats, was that *the excrement of these cats was poisonous to the ground* rendering it sterile and unsupportive of plant life, whereas in the pens of the healthy cats the ground was fertile and supported flourishing vegetation.

Possibly the best examples of the harmful effects of cooked food are the studies of animals in the Philadelphia Zoo by Dr H. Fox, described in his book *Disease in Captive Wild Animals and Birds* (1923). For many years the mortality of animals kept in captivity was very high and attempts to breed them were not very successful. When it was realized that it was false economy to feed animals cheap food such as restaurant scraps etc, and their diets were changed to natural raw foods, straight away the animals' health improved and the mortality rate dropped to very low levels, while at the same time the animals began to breed normally.

Vilhjalmur Stephansson, the Arctic explorer, having observed the splendid health of raw meat-eating Eskimos early this century, adopted an all meat diet with disastrous results, all the worse because of consuming the meat cooked. In admiring their fine health, Stephansson had failed to note that it was short-lived, to be followed by rapid decline and early death. A more recent study of Angmagsalik Eskimos, a community of about 1000 on the east coast of Greenland, showed an average life span of only 27½ years, mainly due to premature degeneration of adults. Their diet consisted of 95% flesh food. The study was by Hoygaard and Pedersen, Copenhagen 1941. This short life span appears to be worse than in the earlier reports on Eskimos elsewhere, and the writer speculates whether the Angmagsalik Eskimos had adopted the practise of cooking their food.

There is an association between the cooking and processing of food and the incidence of cancer, and conversely, it is a fact that cancer patients make the best recoveries on completely raw vegetarian food. In some cases, the reversion to even a partly cooked diet allowed the cancer to re-appear.

This shows that when vital organs are at their lowest state of function, only raw foods make it possible for them to provide the proper body chemistry to maintain health. It follows then, that if raw food permits an otherwise ruined body to restore itself to health, so must raw food provide the maximum benefit to anybody — sick or well.

Cooking and Mutagens

Mutagens are chemicals that can alter the DNA in the nucleus of a living cell so increasing the risk of the cell becoming cancerous. Polynuclear aromatic hydrocarbons (PAH) are such chemicals and it is well known how these may be formed as a result of exposing meat to smoke while cooking it, and of the roasting of coffee. Dr Oliver Alabaster, Associate Professor of Medicine and Director of Cancer Research, George Washington University in his book

What You Can Do to Prevent Cancer (1985) says: "During the past few years it has become apparent that there are many other mutagens beside the PAH's that can be formed by cooking. Most mutagens seem to be formed by an effect of cooking on proteins. This occurs to a greater extent at high temperatures, but can even occur at temperatures below boiling point of water. Broiling hamburgers, beef, fish, chicken, or any other meat, for that matter, will create mutagens, so it appears to be an unavoidable consequence of cooking.

"Other mutagens are formed by the action of cooking on carbohydrates. Even an action as innocent as toasting bread has been shown to create mutagenic chemicals through a process known as the browning reaction. This reaction also occurs when potatoes and beef are fried, or when sugars are heated."

Dr Alabaster went on to describe other mutagens called flavonoids found in tea, coffee, pickles, dill-weed, cocoa, fruit jams, beer, red wine, vinegar, raisins, onions and grape juice.

He continued: "Fortunately, extracts of very few fruits and vegetables are mutagenic. In fact, quite the contrary. Laboratory tests have demonstrated that a number of substances in foods can actually inhibit the action of many mutagens. Anti-mutagenic activity has been shown in extracts of some common vegetables, fruit and spices, including cabbage, broccoli, green pepper, egg plant, shallots, pineapple, apples, ginger and mint leaf."

Raw Food

Dr Max Garten in his book *The Health Secrets of a Naturopathic Doctor* (1967) described how his health had not much improved by becoming a vegetarian, and how this led him to try a completely raw food regimen. He said: "The results were electrifying; within a few days I felt much stronger with a return of my former enthusiasm. Many of my patients whom I had been able to convert to this new diet also reported similar results." Dr Garten observed that putrefactive bacteria in the colon increased not only with the eating of meat but also with the degree of heat used in cooking all food, and with this increase so also did the odiferousness of the stool increase along with the appearance of aches and pains. He said: "It could only be deduced that certain agents in the diet were either missing or had been altered by the heat.

"The respective protein content of the vegetarian diet had also been found to be indicative of changes in the intestinal flora, legumes such as beans, lentils, peas etc. equally contributing to the display of putrefactive changes."

Thus, although vegetarians usually are healthier and outlive meat eaters, they may not maintain very good health or live to a very advanced age if they continually cook their food.

Raw Fruit, the Natural Food of Primates

People become vegetarians to improve their health and extend their lives. Some vegetarians go a step further and consume their food mainly uncooked, while others go even further and limit their diet to fruit, which they claim to be the natural food of man.

Their argument is sound for a number of reasons, but one way or the other, it is a fact that, in reasonable variation, fruit can provide the full complement of all required nutrients in adequate quantities, remembering that the requirements for protein and fat are much lower than generally believed. Therefore, instead of being considered merely an accessory to conventional meals, fruit should be considered in its own right as a staple food. The advantages of a fruitarian diet are:

1. It provides complete nourishment with the minimum of extraneous substances capable of 'silting' up the tissues.
2. It is most easily digested, minimizing the energy required for digestion (which is substantial) thereby minimizing total food (calorie) requirements.
3. It is palatable.
4. It is easily obtained and easily prepared.
5. It satisfies the appetite when sufficient has been eaten —

fruitarians are always lean.
6. Minimum but adequate protein is provided
7. Minimum but adequate essential fats are provided.
8. Maximum energy is available from what is eaten, with only carbondioxide and water, which are entirely non-toxic, as the byproducts.
9. It provides the body with adequate amounts of pure water.
10. It results in a favorable alkaline internal state.
11. Favorable intestinal flora predominate in the bowel.
12. No constipation occurs.
13. No auto-intoxication occurs.
14. The body de-toxifies itself.
15. The blood is clean and low viscosity, there is good circulation with low blood pressure.
16. There is the least wear and tear and the least 'silting up' of all the body organs and tissues.

That fruit, alone, can ideally sustain human health and vigor, even without drinking water, indicates that it indeed provides the basis of man's natural diet. Further substantiation of this view is that there are about forty distinct anatomical, physiological and biological features of humans which show unquestionably that the human body is designed mainly for a fruit diet, notwithstanding the fact that, like all animals, they can survive less successfully on a wide variety of foods. These features range from natural fondness for sweet foods, jaw and teeth structure, salivary secretion, length of digestive tract, size of pancreas, stereo color vision and so on. In fact in all these respects, humans are practically identical today with the more primitive primates in the wild which, whenever possible, live on fruit.

Evidence of the suitability of fruit as a staple food and not just as an accessory to the conventional diet, is to be seen by observing fruitarians who live entirely on a wide variety of fresh fruit, and who display lean, youthful bodies, low blood pressure, clear vision and unimpaired faculties, even with advancing years.

A well known human peculiarity never before connected with this argument but which provides almost conclusive evidence, is that humans, like all primates, are incapable of making Vitamin C in their bodies whereas other animals can (excepting guinea pigs and fruit-eating bats). Basing their argument on this fact, it is strongly advocated by many authorities that people should take large amounts of supplementary Vitamin C to compensate for this 'error of Nature' which they put down to an unfavorable mutation in our evolutionary past some millions of years ago. To prove this argument completely wrong, and at the same time prove that man is a natural fruit eater, consider:

1. The only mutations which persist to become a universal feature of a species are favorable ones. Unfavorable mutations cannot possibly do so.
2. A genetic change preventing the synthesis of vitamin C in the body, to become universal to an entire species, must therefore have been, at the time, a favorable change.
3. The only possibility of such a genetic change being favorable is for the species to have been already getting more than adequate vitamin C, and that any more was undesirable.
4. The only source of 'excess' vitamin C in Nature is a diet of raw fruit. (Only certain tropical fruits contain such high levels of Vitamin C; many fruits contain only small amounts.)

Therefore it is clear that the human diet ideally, should be based mainly on fresh fruit, and that past errors which have led to widespread vitamin C deficiencies are dietary — not genetic — errors.

Obviously some fruits are more nutritious than others, and quality will vary according to the quality of the soil in which they are grown. Commercially grown fruit may contain various levels of insecticide poisons, in which case the fruit should be carefully washed or peeled. At the time of writing, the author has subsisted almost entirely on commercially grown fruit for six years, all the while working long hours under stress seven days a week, and has maintained excellent health. I have chosen the fruit at random* with a preference for tropical fruits, and included dried fruits from time to time without any attempt at being scientific about it. It is claimed by some people that such a diet will eventuate in high blood triglycerides and this is why Nathan Pritikin limited fruit. The increase in triglycerides is supposed to follow elevated levels of blood sugar after eating fruit, but this does not occur with eating whole raw fruit, particularly eaten at whim throughout the day rather than in three large meals. An objection to acid fruits such as citrus and pineapples, particularly if unripe, is that eaten in excess, the acid may cause erosion in the enamel of the teeth. It is interesting to note here that with good body chemistry and a clean mouth, teeth, like bones, are to a great extent self repairable. With half my teeth jammed with fillings, maybe they are beyond self repair, but at my six-monthly pilot medical checkups, I enjoy being told by my doctor I have the arteries and blood pressure of a schoolboy. That makes fruit taste better still, even on a winter's day.

A convert to fruitarianism was the Indian philosopher and statesman Mahatma Gandhi, who after experiencing poor health throughout his youth became a student of Nature Cure at the age of 32. First he became a vegetarian and then a fruitarian. After six months as a fruitarian, he said (quoted from his book *The Health Guide*):

"A period of six months is all too short to arrive at any definite conclusions on such a vital matter as a complete change of diet. This, however, I can say, that, during this period, I have been able to keep well where others have been attacked by disease, and

*It is probably best not to mix the acid fruits with others eaten at the same time. Some people find they experience digestive upsets when at first they embark on a fruitarian diet. This may be because of mixing incompatible fruits or possibly not chewing them properly. The fruit should be taken as snacks throughout the day, as frequently as desired, rather than conventionally as three substantial meals.

If cooked food is eaten at the same time as fruit, the fruit should be eaten first as it digests quickly and clears out of the way of the other food which may reside in the stomach for several hours.

and my physical as well as mental powers are now greater than before. I may not be able to lift heavy loads, but I can do hard labor for a much longer time without fatigue. I can also do more mental work, and with better persistence and resoluteness. I have tried a fruit diet on many sickly people, invariably with great advantage. My own experience, as well as my study of the subject, has confirmed me in the conviction that a fruit diet is the best one for us."

An interesting personality is champion weightlifter, Wiley Brooks, 48, of Venice, California. Most unconventional, Wiley is 6 feet tall and weighs 135 lbs, but can, from a squat rack, lift 935 lbs. He eats only raw fruit and fruit juice.

Dr De Lacy Evans, who devoted most of his professional life to the study of patients, populations, and the factors involved in the aging process, said of fruit:

"There is, therefore, a simplicity, a reason, a wonderful philosophy in the first command given to man — Man may live entirely upon fruits in better health than the majority of mankind now enjoy. Good, sound, ripe fruits are never the cause of disease, but the vegetable acids, as we have before stated, lower the temperature of the body, decrease the process of combustion or oxidation — therefore the waste of the system — less sleep is required, activity is increased, fatigue or thirst is hardly experienced; still the body is well nourished, and as a comparatively small quantity of earthy salts are taken into the system, the cause of old age is in some degree removed, the effect is delayed, and life is prolonged to a period far beyond our 'threescore and ten'."

Water

Water comprises nearly 70% of the body as part of all the tissues and fluids and is constantly being eliminated and replaced. It is eliminated by perspiration and urination and replaced by drinking and eating.

The essence of health being the detoxification of the body, all authorities on nutrition agree on the importance of keeping the kidneys "flushed out". Some authorities insist that you should plan to drink so many glasses of water a day to ensure proper flushing takes place, even if you are not thirsty.

But why can't you rely on your natural senses of feeling thirst to tell you when and how much to drink? The answer is, of course, that you can.

Protein, when eaten, requires seven times more water in its metabolism in the body than does carbohydrate due to the fact so many toxins are produced from protein which must be eliminated in the urine. A high protein diet therefore results in thirst, and the extra water needed is replaced when the thirst is satisfied. The urine is distinctly colored and smelly.

On the other hand, a high carbohydrate diet results in lesser amounts of toxins and little or no thirst is experienced because the byproducts are mainly carbondioxide and pure water. Less urination is required and little if any water need be drunk, unless of course hard work or heat causes more than ordinary perspiration. The urine is only slightly colored.

Fruitarians hardly ever get thirsty. Not only is their diet high in carbohydrate but they of course receive a great deal of water in the juice of the fruit they eat. This water, like the water made in their bodies from the carbohydrate, is absolutely pure. Fruitarians urinate more for the purpose of offloading excess water than for eliminating toxins because so little toxic matter is produced within them other than the normal waste products of their cells. Their urine is clear, odorless, and so is their perspiration.

Hot spices like curry will induce great thirst within minutes of commencing the meal. Should you drink with meals? I speak from experience. On my first trip to Singapore in 1946 I ate the traditional Sunday curry lunch at the old Seaview Hotel. Half way through the meal, perspiration started pouring from me, even from the top of my head. Before I'd finished the main course I had consumed a whole king-sized pitcher of iced water, and without that iced water I think I'd have died of thirst before the dessert course. Can you imagine what pandemonium such foods stir up within you? Salt has the same effect.

It is sometimes insisted that water taken with meals will dilute the digestive juices and impede digestion but this is not so; liquids quickly transit the stomach, bypassing the digesting food there and have little, if any, effect on the process.

Drinking water should be as pure as possible, such as clean rainwater or distilled, because the purpose of water is to dissolve unwanted substances so as to cleanse the tissues as well as dissolve wanted substances and distribute them as part of the blood. Mineral or spring water is more likely to introduce unwanted substances into the body and, one way or another, will not perform as well as pure water.

Summarizing on Human Nutrition

Whereas it is clear that the human body can be reasonably sustained on foods of a widely varying nature — either cooked or raw, high protein or low, high carbohydrate or low, or high fat or low, it would appear that it doesn't matter greatly what sort of food is eaten as long as, one way or another, the needs of the body are provided.

But indeed it does matter how the needs of the body are supplied because some diets, while containing all the necessities, at the same time cause a great deal of harm over varying periods of time.

In the chapter which follows, it is described how the traditional Western diet is responsible for the diseases of civilization which are our major causes of death. This alarming situation has become to some extent recognized by the medical profession which is at last beginning to take an interest in nutrition, but unfortunately the doctors are providing advice based on traditional dietary concepts which are still very much in error.

Despite the fact that the dangers of fat, cholesterol and excess protein have been known for fifty years or more, the mixed diet using foods from the "five main food groups" as recommended by the health authorities today, ensures the intake of these substances in dangerous amounts. As well, the conventional use of salt, sugar, processed starch, alcohol, coffee, tea and condiments is condoned on the principle that "all things in moderation" are OK. Recommended by the British Medical Assocation, the book *Executive Health* by David Carrick, medical supervisor of the English *Financial Times,* advised that life should be enjoyed and that "a little bit of what you fancy does you good."

But what is moderation? Dr Carrick died of a heart attack two years after his book was published.

Therefore whereas following conventional advice about nutrition will usually improve the average person's health, such improvement falls far short of an ideal result.

As we have seen, the traditional so-called balanced diet is hopelessly out of 'balance', and when a lot more man-made indiscretions are added to it — such as salt, cream, oil, sugar, coffee, tea, condiments, candy, soft drinks, alcohol and so on — it becomes a lot worse.

What then is the ideal diet? An ideal diet is one which contains nothing potentially harmful and at the same time contains all the requirements with no deficiencies and no excesses, easy to assimilate with no undue strain on the system, and with residues that are easily expelled from the body. No food of any kind, once cooked, can meet these criteria.

In the jungles of the Philippines, the Japanese soldier refugee would have been — of necessity — on a diet close to the ideal. Probably for the first time in his life his senses of sight, smell and taste gave him accurate advice on what was suitable food because the artificial stimulation provided by cooked, spiced and salted food was not there to deceive them.

In a nutshell, to improve human nutrition the human errors must be eliminated. For best results all the errors must of course be corrected, but this is easier said than done, because hardly anything in our conventional diet is right to start with, a fact which is not fully comprehended by most of the trained so-called experts of nutrition, who continue to promote many unsuitable foods, in moderation, as highly virtuous.

We must adapt our thinking to fit the facts. When it comes to nutrition it's best not to take too many chances. Moderation in all things is, generally speaking, good advice, but advice that can sometimes get you into trouble.

CHAPTER FIVE

The Western Diet — Public Enemy No. 1

"The fact is, there is only one major disease, and that is malnutrition. All ailments and afflictions to which we may become heir are directly traceable to this major disease.

Dr C. W. Cavanaugh, Cornell University

The industrialized nations of the Western World are sometimes referred to as the affluent societies because of their high standards of living. The average life expectancy in these countries has risen significantly over the past hundred years due mainly to improved nutrition in all stratas of society, particularly the working class who have become able to afford food of wider choice and quality. The resultant improved general health has led to diminished infant mortality and greater general resistance to infectious diseases, which benefits are reflected in the life expectancy statistics.

But the Western World still suffers from malnutrition. When malnutrition is mentioned, the thought that comes to mind is the picture of a weak, skinny waif, semi-starved for want of food. But equally malnourished is the rotund wealthy squire dining on roast beef and pheasant; he too suffers from malnutrition and will inevitably die prematurely because of it.

But what of the lean and muscular sportsman? Would you call him malnourished? Ask Arthur Ashe, the Wimbledon tennis champion who had a heart attack at age 34, or one of the many super-fit joggers who have been incapacitated by heart attacks or arthritis.

The malnutrition of the affluent countries of today is insidious and affects everyone to some degree or other — statesmen, workmen, businessmen, film stars, airline pilots, housewives and school kids, and the cause of their malnutrition is the Western diet, the one so fondly prepared by loving wives and mothers at home and by the chefs in the very best restaurants.

The proof of this is revealed by the results of tests which show that even children have elevated cholesterol levels and high blood pressure, as well as the usual tooth decay, pimples and so on. Autopsies of young people killed in accidents show their coronary arteries to be already diseased. Head colds, arthritis and asthma are common, and it is considered normal for blood pressure to increase with age and for people to require reading glasses at age 45. In fact it is almost considered normal to have a heart attack followed by a bypass operation at about age 55. And to cap those 'normal' events off, it is considered normal as well to die around the age of 70 of either a heart attack, stroke or cancer. The lucky ones live a little longer wandering around vaguely in nursing homes until some other form of degeneration catches up with them.

The causes of all these health problems are clearly related to poor body chemistry resulting from bad nutrition, and the proof of this is the rapidity with which most of these problems are reversed when proper dietary correction is employed.

The prefix 'mal' in French means bad. Malnutrition means bad nutrition, not just undernutrition. The integrity of a diet may be impaired in a number of ways:

1. too little food;
2. too much food;
3. lack of essential nutrients, vitamins, minerals;
4. too much protein;
5. too much fat;
6. too much cholesterol;

7. too much starch;
8. too little natural carbohydrate;
9. too little fiber;
10. the use of refined carbohydrates such as flour, sugar, alcohol;
11. the use of salt and condiments;
12. the use of tea, coffee, soft drinks;
13. preservatives in food which upset digestive enzymes;
14. damage to molecular structure of food nutrients caused by heat, particularly deep frying;
15. lack of natural enzymes destroyed by cooking;
16. additives and other chemicals.

The modern diet errs in every one of these factors except the first, and depending on the degree of error, so varies the rate of degeneration within the body. Working hard, the digestive system and other vital organs do their best to maintain a reasonable standard of blood chemistry and so a reasonable standard of health is maintained until the vital organs begin to weaken. Life expectancy varies inversely with the degree of malnutrition which is determined not only by the make-up of the diet but also by the amount consumed, meaning that on the modern 'Western' diet the people who indulge sparingly of it suffer less degeneration and so live longer.

By comparing the make-up of the typical Western diet with the natural diet upon which the human race evolved, and upon which in the Philippine jungle the Japanese soldier escaped the diseases of civilization, we can more clearly see the major errors that compound the health of modern people.

	Natural Diet	*Western Diet*
Calories for adult male approx.	2000	3500
Vitamin C approx.	3000-9000 mg	100 mg
Other vitamins and minerals	adequate	?
Natural enzymes	ideal	almost nil
Protein % approx.	4% (ideal)	15% (hazardous)
Fat % approx.	4% (ideal)	40% (dangerous)

	Natural Diet	*Western Diet*
Natural carbohydrate % approx.	92% (ideal)	5% (inadequate)
Refined carbohydrate % approx.	nil	40% (dangerous)
Cholesterol	almost nil	400 mg (dangerous)
Fiber	adequate	inadequate
Salt and condiments	nil	hazardous
Caffeine in tea, coffee, soft drinks	nil	hazardous
Preservatives	nil	hazardous
Heat damage to food	nil	hazardous
Chemicals	nil	hazardous

These comparisons tell the story. The so-called balanced diet with its animal protein of meat, chicken, eggs, fish and dairy products, contains what amounts to, over the years, lethal quantities of fat, cholesterol and protein — the subtances most directly associated with every one of the metabolic and degenerative diseases.

Fat is without doubt the most dangerous of all dietary substances. In Nature the diet of most primates would scarcely amount to 4% fat. New Guinea highlanders live in good health on a diet containing 4% fat. Years of research led Nathan Pritikin to place an absolute limit of 10% fat in the diet. And yet people, day after day, year after year, consume food containing over four times Pritikin's limit and nine times Nature's ideal, and then on top of that many double that again by eating twice as much food as they need! No wonder arteries get blocked with fat and cholesterol!

Examine the pictures of red blood cells on page 80. See how the cells of normal blood look and compare how they look when all stuck together with fat. And that's only the red cells; the blood platelets which are smaller and not visible in the photo, clump together too, the clear blood serum is also sticky of course and so is the vital fluid, lymph, which bathes the body's cells. No wonder the heart pumps harder to increase the blood pressure, it's a wonder the circulation flows at all. with red blood cells stuck together and with impaired circulation, the oxygen supply to the

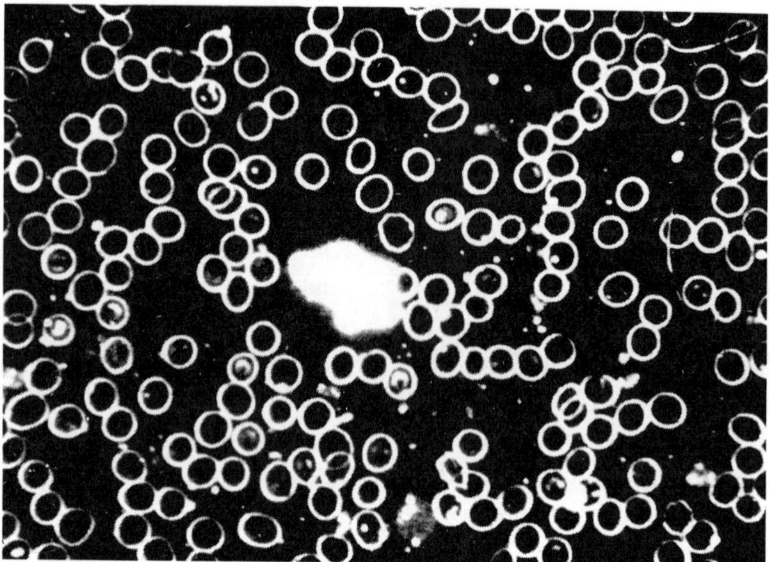

Dark field high power view of normal non-aggregation red blood cells six hours after a low-fat meal.

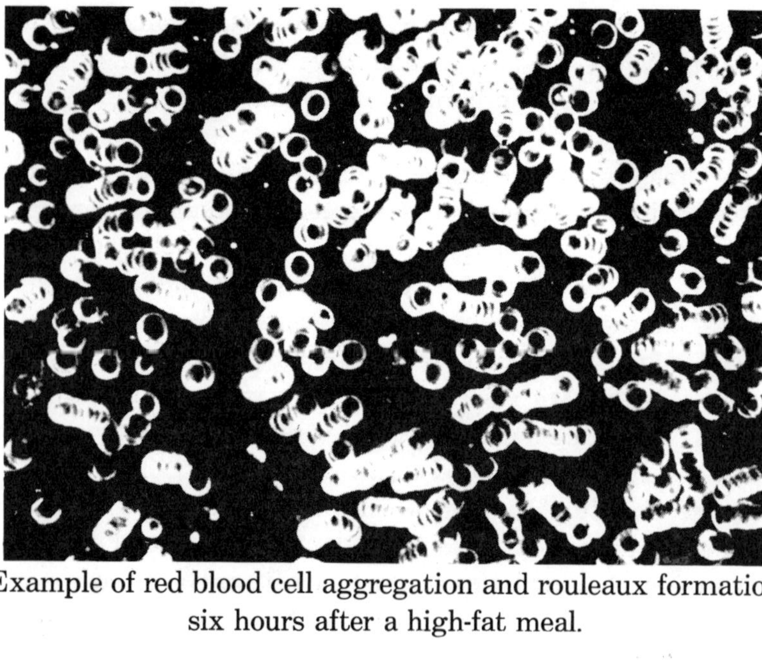

Example of red blood cell aggregation and rouleaux formation six hours after a high-fat meal.

tissues is depleted. What chance then for healthy cells and a properly functioning brain and body?

Cholesterol is probably the next most dangerous dietary substance. Absolute vegetarian animals, such as rabbits, have no means of processing cholesterol at all in their bodies and when fed a diet containing cholesterol their arteries rapidly fill with it and they die. Humans are capable of coping with about 100 milligrams of cholesterol per day from cooked food without suffering artery disease, but the Western diet's high levels (up to maybe 800 mg) is a guarantee of heart disease and choked up arteries elsewhere in the body. Eskimos, whose diet consists mainly of meat and fat high in cholesterol, nevertheless exhibit low levels of it in their blood and do not suffer from atherosclerosis to the extent that would be expected from such a diet. Nor are high levels of ketones exhibited which would normally be expected from all the fat. This is because the enzymes in their uncooked food enable the body to more thoroughly break down the fat and cholesterol. Similarly, wild animals whose diets are exclusively raw meat and fat exhibit perfectly healthy arteries at all times.

Protein in excess of the body's requirements is a disease producing factor by virtue of the toxic byproducts formed as a residue of its metabolism in the body, as has already been explained. High protein diets, particularly diets high in meat, are associated consistently with not only heart disease, but cancer, arthritis, osteoporosis and kidney failure. Although the animal protein foods contribute most to the excess of protein in the Western diet, some vegetables such as beans, peas, soya beans and other lentils contain substantial amounts, and so too do cereals, particularly some types of wheat. All of these protein sources are unnecessary because adequate amounts of protein exist in simple fruit and vegetables.

When the body's need for food is mainly for fuel to supply energy, and when the food most safely and easily converted for this purpose is natural carbohydrate, it is purposeless and dangerous to load the body up with over half its intake of food in the form of protein and fat with only 45% as carbohydrate — most of which in the modern diet is in the form of starch and refined sugar, high in calories but low in nutritive value.

Salt is used as a food preservative and performs this function by virtue of the fact it inhibits the action of enzymes. Thus salt places strain on the digestive system as well as being a powerful irritant capable of destroying cells in the sensitive lining of the mouth and digestive tract. Salt is suspected as an accessory to stomach cancer because of this irritating effect.

Condiments too are irritants with no food value and enter the body only to be expelled via the kidneys, which on the Western diet are already overworked by the protein and fat residues. The intake of large amounts of curry and Worcestershire sauce is known to produce kidney disease, commonly referred to as 'Curry Kidney' and 'Worcestershire Sauce Kidney'.

The lack of fiber in the Western diet ensures that most people have constipation, which is a condition accepted as part of life, along with head colds, arthritis and so on, and most households are well stocked with laxatives along with aspirin and dozens of other pills and poisons. People who refuse to use laxatives have two options left: they can ladle bran* flakes onto their fiberless food, or keep a supply of magazines in the bathroom. Along with constipation come piles (haemhorroids) and hernias. As is explained in the next chapter, constipation is not merely an inconvenience, it is probably the most potent contributor to toxemia of the blood stream and is associated with all kinds of cancer, particularly, of course, cancer of the bowel.

Heat damage to the constituents in food and the destruction of the more fragile enzymes are faults not only with the Western diet but with the diets of people everywhere, and alone are responsible for increasing the workload on the digestive system

***Bran.* The idea of adding bran flakes to food is to add fiber to fiber-deficient food and so avoid constipation. Bran, however, does not act in the same fashion as natural vegetable fiber but acts more as an irritant, and as such is capable of damaging the delicate mucous membrane lining the digestive tract.

and vital organs so that hardly a person on Earth manages to attain the full potential of their life. The lifespan of Eskimos is even briefer than most because notwithstanding their practise of eating their food mainly raw, their enormous intake of protein and fat ensures rapid degeneration of their bodies with subsequent early onset of old age and decrepitude.

I'll not go into a discussion on the quality of food and the merits of organically grown vegetables etc. other than to say that organically grown food must be considered superior only providing that the soil in which it is grown is complete to start with. The fact that food is produced 'organically' is not a guarantee that it provides perfect nutrition. The quality of food is a factor of utmost importance but is a subject outside our terms of reference which must be confined to improving our nutrition with better understanding of how to use the materials already available to us.

I shall conclude this chapter with a reference to 'fast', 'take-away' foods. In *The Health Revolution* is a more detailed discussion on these foods which can be summed up by saying that due to the method of preparation, high heat, fat, salt, cholesterol and refined carbohydrate and other dangerous factors, these sorts of foods are more dangerous than the home-cooked versions of the Western way of eating and that the increased use of them, particularly when they are washed down with cola and other junk drinks, must inevitably accelerate the decline in the health of modern society.

'New' viruses and 'new' diseases are being discovered almost every day. They 'threaten' mankind but curiously leave animals alone. The explanation for this is obvious — don't blame the viruses and germs, they've been around for thousands of millions of years; they are opportunistic and 'attack' only organisms that are weak and defective. This is a simple fact of life (and death) which becomes more and more evident as the Western diet becomes more and more unnatural.

CHAPTER SIX

Toxemia and the Diseases of Civilization

"I know of nothing so potent in maintaining good health in laboratory animals as perfectly constituted food; I know of nothing so potent in producing ill health as improperly constituted food. This, too, is the experience of stock breeders. Is man an exception to a rule so universally applicable to the higher animals?"

Major General Sir Robert McCarrison M.D.

Doctor John Tilden in his book, *Toxemia Explained*, said there are over 400 catalogued diseases listed in medical text books. That was in 1926; who knows how many are listed today? Every one of these diseases however, Dr Tilden explained, is merely a symptom of some sort of organic malfunction caused by toxemia in the blood.

As already described, the health of the entire body is dependent on the condition of the *Milieu Interieur*, or in other words, the condition of the blood and lymph fluid. With few exceptions, diseases of any kind only occur when fat, cholesterol and various toxic substances derived from improper diet enter the circulation to upset the body chemistry and to deplete the oxygen available to the body's cells. Dr Tilden was merely restating the earlier concept of Professor Claude Bernard and Professor Antoine Bechamp when he said there was only one disease — not hundreds — and this was toxemia, which disrupted normal metabolism and at the same time reduced the body's resistance to germs.

Nathan Pritikin said exactly the same thing but added the prefix 'lipo' (meaning fat) to coin the name lipotoxemia, to emphasize the fact that fat in the blood was the worst disease factor of them all.

The different manifestations of disease have all been medically classified according to the symptoms displayed. There are Metabolic diseases, Degenerative diseases, Deficiency diseases, Mental diseases, Infectious diseases, and so on, but as 'Nature Cure' doctors all agree, the scientific name and classification is not important because the only form of treatment effective in all cases is to restore the proper internal milieu whereupon the body restores itself to normal function without further help. The capability of the body, given favorable circumstances, to heal and restore itself is astonishing, but when vital organs have become degenerated beyond repair or when cancer has progressed beyond a certain stage, it may of course be too late for the body to make a come-back.

Although there are no races of people in the world who are completely free of disease of some kind due to the fact that diets everywhere are defective in one way or another, the widest variety of diseases, most of them unknown among primitive natives, is to be found in the highly 'civilized' countries which are the industrialized nations of the Western world. Doctors who over the past hundred years have served in remote uncivilized areas have consistently observed the absence among the natives of cancer, heart disease, stroke and all other forms of circulatory disease, hypertension, arthritis, multiple sclerosis, asthma, diabetes, pre-menstrual tension, migraine, prostatitis, glaucoma and many others which are common in civilization.

When primitive natives adopt the white man's food, they soon begin to exhibit the symptoms of the white man's diseases. The good news is that when the white man adopts the diet of the primitive natives the symptoms of his civilized diseases soon diminish and go away. The Japanese are not primitive people but until World War II were more or less isolated from the Western world with different customs and a traditional diet based on rice, seafood and vegetables, almost all of it cooked. Heart disease and cancer incidence (except for stomach cancer) was low, compared to that in the Western world where these diseases account for the majority of deaths.

Before World War II however, many Japanese migrated to the USA and it was observed that after a few years of becoming Americanized and adopting American eating habits the migrants began to display the same diseases common in America. Since WWII the entire Japanese nation has become more and more Americanized and as a result the rate of heart disease etc. has steadily increased. A prominent Japanese doctor, speaking in America not long ago, said he had looked out from a hotel window in Tokyo recently and noticed a large neon sign in the form of a big M and had remarked to himself that Japan's retribution for WWII had finally arrived. The good doctor will have something to freak right out on when the fried chicken and pizza palaces get going in Japan!

It is not within the scope of this book to explain the common "diseases of civilization" and how they are individually caused; that has already been done in *The Health Revolution.* Sufficient be it to repeat that diagnosis and specialized treatment of the common complaints of today — and indeed the uncommon ones too — are completely unnecessary when all that is required is to correct the diet and perhaps other bad lifestyle habits and stand clear. The healing power of Nature does the rest.

However, because of the continuing devastation to our society by heart disease and cancer, the threat now posed by our new star turn AIDS, and the increasing nuisance of the common cold and arthritis, a brief discussion of these now follows.

HEART DISEASE AND STROKE

Heart disease, together with strokes, account for about 50% of all deaths in the Western countries. The disease is caused by the gradual blocking of arteries with fat and cholesterol, a 'mushy' condition called atherosclerosis which starts in early childhood and advances relentlessly throughout life. Even on a diet low in fat and cholesterol but very high in grain products, artery disease of a different nature can occur in which the artery walls harden with calcium and gradually close. Once upon a time, this hardening of the arteries was more common than mushy atheroma, and was referred to as arteriosclerosis, but nowadays with so much fat and cholesterol in the diet, atherosclerosis is the condition almost universal.

All arteries are affected, not only the coronary arteries of the heart. The condition may interrupt blood flow to the brain and cause a stroke, or to the legs and cause claudication, or to the kidneys and cause kidney failure. Eyesight, hearing and mental faculties become diminished, and the whole body deteriorates. Regardless of which part of the body first begins to exhibit symptoms of distress, it must be realized that the disease has been building up, unsuspectedly, for many years in all parts of the body, and if permitted to continue will inevitably result in premature death, unless of course cancer intervenes first.

It is clear then that atherosclerosis (or arteriosclerosis), the direct result of improper diet, accounts in the first place for a substantial proportion of the hundreds of separately defined diseases of civilization. Fortunately atherosclerosis is a reversible process, even from a very advanced stage, once the proper dietary corrections have been made, and of course so too are the so-called diseases associated with it. World War II provided good evidence of this when in Europe meat, dairy products and sugar became very scarce and death rates from heart disease and cancer fell dramatically.

The solution to the problem of heart disease is simple. Just stop eating the things that cause it.

CANCER

Cancer is not a fearsome entity of unknown origin that wears a hundred different masks and strikes wantonly at innocent people, as is commonly believed. Fearsome it may be, but mysterious not at all. It is an absolutely normal biological process which occurs as a consequence of certain changes to the environment of perfectly normal cells of the body, a process which has been demonstrated many times in scientific experiments. Dr Otto Warburg (the recipient of two Nobel Prizes), and a number of other researchers, described the process of cancer clearly many years ago, but unfortunately the medical profession, displaying a lamentable lack of comprehension, still regards cancer as a fearsome intruder to be destroyed with the harshest of measures.

Be that as it may, even blind Freddie can see that when cancer kills 25% of civilized people while among some less civilized populations the disease is unknown, the civilized people must be doing something very wrong. Very wrong indeed, because the uncivilized people don't get heart disease either. And as we shall see, like heart disease and the other diseases of civilization, cancer is not only very simply avoidable, but in many cases reversible by purely natural means.

Here's where we get back to the subject of pure blood and healthy cells.

How good is your memory? Do you recall from chapter 2 the difference between a primitive cell and a differentiated cell? How cells get oxygen and nutrients from the lymph fluid that flows by them? Understanding these things is the key to understanding cancer. The description which now follows is a composite of the research findings of a great number of physicians and bio-chemists who, over the past one hundred years, have studied cancer both in the laboratory and in the human body. It is much abbreviated of course, and is more fully dealt with in *The Health Revolution.*

Understanding cancer

When bacteria, which are single cell organisms, are deprived of oxygen they are capable of survival by reverting to the process of fermentation of nutrients in order to produce the energy they need. This process, called glycolysis, was the process used by primitive cells billions of years ago before oxygen became freely available in the sea and air, and is still part of the aerobic respiratory process employed by oxygen-using cells of living creatures today.

Glycolysis is an inefficient process which liberates only small amounts of energy from a given amount of blood sugar, leaving a residue of pyruvic acid which is converted to lactic acid and eliminated. Oxygen-using (aerobic) cells still retain glycolysis in the initial stages of their respiratory cycle but are immensely more efficient because they are capable of taking the pyruvic acid resultant from glycolysis and combining it with oxygen, which process not only liberates about fifteen times more energy but at the same time leaves only carbondioxide and water as byproducts, substances which are completely harmless and easily eliminated.

In order to survive by fermentation, aerobic bacteria must change into a more primitive form, and because fermentation is so inefficient, more carbohydrate (food) must be consumed and a lot of acid produced. This process occurs in the mouth when the natural bacteria there are deprived of oxygen by food residues stuck between the teeth, and the acid so produced eats away the tooth enamel to make the cavities we call tooth decay. Similarly, aerobic bacteria normal in the colon (bowel) change into anaerobic bacteria when putrifying residues of protein and fat cause constipation, and acids and other toxins are produced, many of which find their way into the bloodstream.

When lipotoxemia and acidic conditions of the blood result in deterioration of the lymph which sustains the tissue cells of the body, the cells may be deprived of oxygen or deprived of the enzymes they need to utilize oxygen. When this occurs the *milieu interiur,* polluted, is referred to as the Cancer Milieu.

Like bacteria (which are cells) the cells of the human body are similarly capable of reverting to a more primitive form when forced to by interference to their normal respiration, and the more their aerobic respiration is curtailed, the more primitive they must become in order to survive. Thus for a normal fully differentiated cell — e.g. a lung cell — to change into a more primitive form it must de-differentiate, and in degrees lose its identity as a lung cell, and resemble more and more the primitive embryo cells from which the body originated. The degree of de-differentiation is proportional to the degree the cell is dependent on fermentation to survive, and when the cell reaches a certain stage of primitiveness it forgets its allegiance to the body as a whole and starts to reproduce as primitive cells do, heedless of the body's normal constraints. This unrestrained growth of de-differentiated cells is cancer, and the tumor at the site of origin is called the primary tumor.

The degree of de-differentiation determines the primitiveness of the cells and therefore their rate of growth, which means that the malignancy of the cancer is directly related to the degree of de-differentiation, fermentation and production of lactic acid. Thus the cancer growth proceeds in a vicious circle because the lactic acid and other waste products of the cancer cells worsen further the Cancer Milieu which started the process off in the first place. Moreover, because the cancer cells resemble embryonic cells in structure and function they are capable of producing the same blocking factor embryonic cells do, which inhibits the immune system from attacking them.

Cells do not have to be fully de-differentiated to grow as cancer and therefore pathology tests can usually identify them with the tissue of their origin. Thus when cancer cells migrate in the blood and lymph and start secondary tumors elsewhere in the body, the site of the primary growth can usually be determined by examination of cells from the secondary. The secondary growths are the most fast-growing because although at the tissue of their origin the normal constraints to growth still tend to control the primary cancer, away from the tissue of origin the constraints do not exist.

As the vicious circle of cancer growth proceeds, more and more of the body's supply of blood sugar is squandered in the wasteful production of lactic acid and so the entire body, starved of sustenance, wastes away in the condition known as cachexia.

The major factor underlying the cancer process is improper diet. The incidence of all kinds of cancer is related more to the high intake of cooked food containing fat, protein, cholesterol, salt and preservatives than to anything else, although anything at all detrimental to the purity of the bloodstream must one way or another contribute to the problem. The deprivation of oxygen to the cells is caused not only by high blood viscosity, poor circulation and low oxygen levels, but also by the absence of the enzymes required to complete the respiratory cycle even when oxygen is available. The respiratory enzymes may be absent because of nutrients missing from the diet, or the respiratory enzymes may be inhibited by carcinogens in the bloodstream derived from sources such as food, smoking, alcohol, putrefaction in the colon, and poisons from infected teeth.

Dr Joseph Issels of Germany who has researched and treated cancer for fifty years asserts that poisoning from infected teeth is one of the prime causes of cancer, and this viewpoint is supported by Dr Mulhim Hassan of Lebanon in his book *Prevention and Cure of Cancer.*

The cancer process, like atherosclerosis, takes many years to develop, and the onset of the cancer growth itself usually appears in middle age or later when the vital organs have degenerated to the stage they can no longer maintain a reasonable degree of purity of the *milieu interieur.* In the years preceding the appearance of cancer as a growth, the tissues pass through a stage known as pre-cancer, and while the body's immune system is capable of reasonable function, any cancer cells that form, at least in the early stages, may be quickly destroyed by the immune system's white cells, providing of course that the white cells are capable of reasonable function. It should be noted that fat and cholesterol in the blood severely inhibit the white cells' activity.

Primary cancer occurs mainly in tissues which in their day to day function have a constant wearing out and renewal of cells — tissues such as the skin, the lining of the digestive tract, the respiratory tract and the female genital canal. Apart from the fact that the cells in these tissues tend to rapidly reproduce anyway, these tissues are exposed to irritation of various kinds which promotes normal renewal growth. New growth requires temporary de-differentiation of cells in any tissue, and if the tissue is in a pre-cancerous state any irritation or injury may be sufficient to trigger partially de-differentiated cells into becoming cancer cells. It has been postulated in the past that irritation or injury may be a cause of cancer, a postulation which of course is incorrect because irritation or injury cannot trigger cancer in healthy tissue.

Cancer is often also linked with emotional factors such as worry and grief. The two factors, injury and stress, time and again precede the appearance of cancer, separately or together, and have often been thought to be primary causes of cancer. However it is clear that cancer occurs only in tissue that is pre-cancerous beforehand and that irritation and emotional stress are only secondary factors, irritation by its effect on triggering cell growth, and emotional stress by its effect on depressing the cancer-fighting ability of the body's immune system. Hormone imbalance may also enter the picture; breast cancer is often associated with high levels of estrogen, the female growth hormone, and it should be noted that over-production of estrogen is caused by high levels of fat in the diet. Smoking is considered to be the primary cause of lung cancer but research has shown that its role in producing lung cancer is mainly that of an irritant triggering new growth in tissue already pre-cancerous. Asbestos causes similar irritation. The role of smoking as a real primary cancer cause is its effect of introducing carbon monoxide into the bloodstream and reducing available oxygen to the tissues. Strong sunshine is thought to be the prime cause of skin cancer but it is no such thing; it is an irritant which triggers new cell growth it is true, but skin cancer only eventuates in skin which is pre cancerous, and when people adopt a low fat, low cholesterol diet they find the skin cancers no longer occur.

Billions and billions of dollars have been spent on desperate research to find a cure for cancer, a quest doomed to failure from the start even though doctors talk about various rates of cures obtained by surgery, radiation and chemotherapy. A person is regarded as cured of cancer if after the operation the cancer does not re-appear in five years, and all through that anxious five years or in the next maybe less anxious five years (if the patient lasts that long) nobody knows if and when the cancer will 'strike' again.

Cancer can be considered 'cured' only if the causes underlying it are understood and permanently removed. The simple solution to the cancer problem is to stop doing the things that cause cancer.

AIDS

Viruses and germs existed on planet Earth a couple of billion years before the appearance of human beings. All through the countless ages as the higher forms of life evolved, viruses and germs were all around, but the animal kingdom was untroubled by them because all animals have virus and germ proof bodies. Had their bodies not been virus and germ proof from the start no higher forms of life would have evolved at all. We would not be here.

The hardy forebears of modern man knew nothing of viruses and germs, they too had bodies proofed against them. Woe betide any virus or germ that somehow found its way inside the human body; the powerful white cells of the human immune system would quickly despatch them forever.

So having endured all sorts of incredible hardships in the course of his ascendancy, man had proven his body to be almost indestructible, and this is the same body with which we are all equipped still today. When the need arises, the human body can perform the most herculean tasks, traverse by foot burning deserts and icy wastes, or climb the steepest, highest, frozen mountains, with endurance surpassing that of all other creatures. That is — healthy bodies can, and they don't 'catch' cold doing it, either.

Why is it then that germs and viruses cause so much distress to humans today, while seemingly to leave animals alone? Indeed, why do some people go through life without a day's sickness while others have something always wrong with them? Why do some supposedly healthy folk catch head colds at the drop of a hat while others remain free of them? The answer, of course, is that some people are more prone to sickness than others, and the reason for their proneness is not that they were born that way, it is because their once-sound bodies have degenerated and their natural defenses against disease are only partially working.

Pestilence and disease have always been the major causes of death for mankind, at least as far back as recorded history shows, but the same history reveals that for all that time, malnutrition was almost universal, at least in the civilized countries. The great plagues and epidemics of the past wiped out millions of people, sometimes decimating entire populations, and yet many individuals exposed to the same germs and viruses escaped unscathed. The story is always the same — the poor, underfed and malnourished die like flies while the well-nourished survive.

When germs and viruses were discovered by medical science, it was thought that the cause of all human disease had been found at last. Germs and viruses were enemies to be destroyed. And when antibiotic drugs were invented that wiped out germs and saved people from death by tuberculosis and pneumonia, it seemed that medical science was on the right track.

But antibiotics don't destroy viruses — only germs (including friendly normal bacteria) — so medical science continues desperately to develop vaccines to combat viruses.

Infectious diseases, both germ-related and virus-related, have become more and more common in recent years, the most troublesome being the viral ones. The common cold is more common than ever, and herpes and candidiasis, once uncommon, are now common. The Center for Disease Control in the USA reports that syphilis is increasing "dramatically". Now we have a new virus, the so-called AIDS virus, to 'attack' the human race.

But why only humans? Why aren't animals — whose bodies work the same way as ours, whose immune systems are the same — why aren't they attacked by influenza, herpes and AIDS? Could it be for the same reason they are not 'attacked' by heart disease, cancer and arthritis?

Is it mere coincidence that the Center for Disease Control reports the increased new syphilis cases are mostly among intravenous drug users in areas where AIDS is most common? Are the agents of disease suddenly becoming more powerful, or is it just that the health and fabric of society is disintegrating more rapidly?

It is as clear as the nose on your face that along with the rest of the so-called diseases of civilization, AIDS is a self-inflicted condition. Self-inflicted, not because a person chooses to risk exposure to the 'AIDS virus', but because of indulgence in dietary and other lifestyle habits that enervate their bodies in the first place. A degenerated, run-down, malnourished body is a slowly dying body, offering an open invitation to invasion by any germ or virus happening by. People do not catch AIDS any more than they catch influenza. A vigorously healthy person can be sneezed all over with influenza viruses all day and not 'catch' influenza, but after a spell of too much work and a few late nights, bingo! the same person gets the 'flu. If he is really healthy his immune system will revive quickly after a good rest and banish the 'flu in a day. Due to the Western diet most people's immune systems are depleted in varying degrees all the time, and a cold may last a week or two, or even longer. But do they ever realize the extent that fat and cholesterol inhibits the power of their defensive white cells? Do they ever realize how stress impairs their thymus gland and further reduces their immunocompetence? No, they blame the entire miserable experience on a virus, and if the virus can be traced back to Hong Kong or Timbuctu, their argument sounds even better.

Everybody, everywhere, displays in their blood countless antibodies, a different one for every infection they have ever had in life. Every type of cold virus they have ever encountered — even without having at the time displayed symptoms — will be represented by its own specific antibodies. The antibodies are there to mount an attack if ever the same virus is again encountered. For every person displaying what is colorfully known today as 'full-blown' AIDS, there are hundreds of healthy or fairly healthy people — male and female, heterosexual and homosexual — who test 'HIV antibody positive' meaning that at some time or other in the past the HIV virus has entered their body and that their body has resisted the virus and made antibodies against it should it be again encountered. The Centre for Disease Control (CDC) in the USA stated that in 1985 only one or two per cent of people who tested AIDS positive had developed to be AIDS patients.

As long as good living habits and diet are maintained, a person with AIDS antibodies will remain as healthy as ever, although they will carry the HIV antibodies in their bloodstream, along with all the others, until they die, all the while protected against all viruses and germs by a strong immune system. On the other hand, should their bodies still be harboring the HIV virus, and should they allow their health to decline by following poor dietary habits, smoking, drug taking and further depleting their vitality with sexual excesses and so on, then, as predicted, they will decline and die, all the while blaming their bad luck and the HIV virus.

The cancer 'virus'

For many years research doctors have described the proliferation of virus-like micro-organisms in the tissues and cells of chronically sick people, particularly in the blood and tissues of cancer patients. At one time it was thought that this virus may be the actual cause of cancer. Dr Virginia Livingstone of San Diego has worked for many years to develop a vaccine to destroy this micro-organism she calls 'Progenitor Cryptocides'* and so accelerate the good results she gets by dietary methods. However, it is clear that the proliferation of the cancer 'virus' is only a secondary effect in the degenerative process which leads to cancer, and this is the opinion of most leading researchers including Dr Cornelius Moerman of Holland, probably the most experienced cancer researcher in the world. As Dr Livingstone herself describes in *The Conquest of Cancer* (1984), the Progenitor Cryptocides resides quiescently in the bodies of all people, even new-born babies, just as does the herpes virus; and like herpes, only proliferates with the onset of chronic ill health and the accompanying diminution of the immune system.

So, with AIDS, which came first, the sickness or the virus? The chicken or the egg? The virus originally identified in AIDS patients is called the HTLV-III virus, but since then other similar viruses have been reported. Dr Robert Gallo of the National Cancer Institute thinks that others may yet be discovered. In view of this situation, the virus is referred to now simply as the HIV virus meaning 'Human Immunodeficiency Virus'.

Dr Anthony Morris, another leading virologist, says that "AIDS has been around for years" and that the antibody was identified in blood which had been stored on ice for over forty years. Similarly, the primary symptoms which characterize AIDS:

*These minute virus-like micro-organisms normally exist within all healthy cells, including sperm cells, embryo cells and those of a new-born baby. Dr Livingstone says the so-called viruses, sometimes called C-particles or L-forms, are in fact extremely small microbes similar to the bacilli of tuberculosis and leprosy, and that they form an essential part of the cells of all animals, their function being the production of the growth hormone choriogonadotropin.

Kaposi's sarcoma and pneumo-cystiscarinii are not new diseases, and nor is the practise of homosexual sex.

For hundreds of years, cancer and heart disease were uncommon causes of death but they were known, even though not understood. Just as cancer and heart disease are biological consequences of poor lifestyle and diet it becomes clear that so too is AIDS which is new only to the extent that it is becoming more common and has a virus of its own upon which the blame can be heaped.

Summarizing AIDS

People displaying the disease symptoms collectively known as AIDS come from all strata of society and may be male, female, heterosexual or homosexual. The majority of these people are either homosexuals or malnourished heterosexuals, the majority of the latter being from poverty stricken third world populations.

There have always been homosexual people, but many modern 'liberated' groups lead a lifestyle outrageous to their bodies which includes drug taking, smoking, alcohol, sexual excesses, and the worst features of the Western diet. Even young bodies cannot long stand such abuse; the signs of degeneration soon appear: the vitality of the body and general metabolism diminish, the immune system loses function, and the body — prematurely aged and open for invasion by sundry opportunistic germs and viruses — gradually dies. Blood tests during these proceedings reveal the presence or perhaps only the suspected presence of the HIV virus, AIDS is diagnosed, the patient told he is doomed and so with shattered morale and accepting death as inevitable, he dies on schedule. And all the while this tragedy is being enacted, billions of research dollars are being spent in a futile quest to develop a vaccine, when the answer to the problem is already clear when a little logic is employed.

An article on AIDS by medical writer, Gary Null in *Penthouse* Magazine, called 'AIDS: Don't Panic' hopefully will stimulate some medical logic. In the article, Null reasons: "If only one to two percent of HIV infected people are developing AIDS, there may be good lifesaving medical reasons why the other 98 per cent are not. After all, AIDS is a failure of the immune system to fend off a host of secondary, 'opportunistic' diseases that have been around for centuries. If more and more viruses are discovered to be triggering this breakdown, might it not be that *the **real cause** of AIDS is the **breakdown** itself?*

The good news

When, under medical treatment, the symptoms of a disease regress and disappear the doctor is said to have 'cured' the patient. When the symptoms regress and disappear of their own accord without medical treatment, a disease is said to have gone into 'spontaneous remission'. In both cases however, the recovery is achieved by the self-healing properties of the body itself and usually would have happened whether medicine was used or not.

As we have seen, in order for the self-healing properties of the body to function effectively, the bloodstream must be cleared of toxins and fat — the *milieu interiur* must be purified. There is no metabolic disease that will not rapidly clear once this is done; there is no degenerative disease that will not be slowed and in most cases, reversed. If mental stress can at the same time be removed and the patient given confidence that survival is possible, then the healing process will proceed at a faster rate.

AIDS is no exception to this rule. The blind fear of viruses and germs must give way to logic and understanding. Remember Louis Pasteur's dying words: "Bernard was right. The microbe is nothing, the soil (*milieu interieur*) is everything."

A doctor who has put the concepts of natural healing to good effect in 'curing' AIDS is Dr Ian Brighthope of Melbourne, who has been treating 28 patients over a three year period using dietary methods supplemented with vitamin C and other vitamins and minerals. The 28 patients included eight who had 'full-blown' AIDS and all had shown impressive improvement. His paper on the subject which appeared in the *International Clinical Nutrition Review*, April 1987, is entitled 'AIDS — Remissions using Nutrient Therapies and Megadose Intravenous Ascorbate'.

Other cases have been reported in which very rapid recoveries were obtained using a raw vegetarian diet, sunshine and rest, with no dietary supplements at all.

In the conclusion to his *Penthouse* article, Gary Null described interviews with some hundreds of male homosexuals in which their lifestyle habits were examined. Two groups were interrogated. In the group where lifestyles included high stress, drugs and poor diet, it was found that almost 90% had tested positive for HIV or had AIDS-related complex, or the AIDS antibody, whereas in the group comprised of over 100 vegetarians who abstained from recreational drugs and excessive sexual contact, no symptoms of AIDS could be found.

Nothing could be clearer or simpler — if you don't want AIDS, just stop doing the things that cause it. A healthy body fears no virus, it destroys them in its stride.

ARTHRITIS

Medical authorities say there are many different kinds of arthritis and that the disease is so complex it can only be treated by highly trained specialists and even then is virtually incurable.

Utter nonsense. No matter in how many forms arthritis may present itself, there are only three major factors involved, two of them of dietary origin and the third one being stress. The dietary factors are blood fats and uric acid.

Arthritis has been suspected as being an 'auto-immune' disease, one in which the white cells of the body actually attack the body 'by mistake'. White cells indeed are involved but, like germs, they are being blamed for mistakes made by the person who owns the body, who chooses to live on a high-fat, high-protein diet.

The white cells are of different kinds, the phagocytes being the ones which engulf foreign substances, germs etc., and destroy them with their powerful, corrosive, digestive juices. These white cells constantly patrol the tissues and joints of the body looking for any trouble-makers.

Arthritis is caused in two ways. When, due to high fat levels in the blood and poor circulation, the oxygen level in the synovial fluid which lubricates the joints becomes so low that the white cells in that location perish, the cells disintegrate, and when they disintegrate their corrosive digestive juices attack the joint and damage it. That is osteoarthritis. Gouty arthritis occurs the same way except that in this case the white cells are destroyed by crystals of uric acid which precipitate in the blood mainly as a result of eating too much protein. Uric acid is normal in the blood in small quantities in solution but on a high protein diet the concentration becomes so great that crystals are precipitated, and these are needle-sharp so when ingested by the white cells the cells are punctured and destroyed. High blood fat levels exacerbate the uric acid problem by virtue of the fact they impede the clearance of the acid from the bloodstream.

The two processes of course may occur simultaneously and will be exacerbated by stress which causes an increase in blood fats and blood viscosity. Bread, alcohol and refined sugar are other exacerbating factors. The calcium build-up which occurs at the joints is due to the body's efforts of self-protection when calcium is taken from the bones to counteract the high acid levels. Herein, of course, lies the cause of osteoporosis, the disease in which the bones become de-calcified.

Rheumatism occurs when tissues other than the joints are affected by the same destructive processes that cause arthritis.

So it can be seen that arthritis, rheumatism and osteoporosis present no greater mystery than heart disease, multiple sclerosis, cancer and all the rest. If you get your diet right, and correct your other living habits you will not only not require the services of a 'specialist' who specializes in giving advice that does not work, but you will only need your doctor on the occasions when you are injured in some hazardous form of healthy, physical activity.

The Pritikin diet and arthritis

A special word of warning is necessary to those who follow the Pritikin diet. As I have already described from personal experience and from the experience of many others, the Pritikin diet is acid forming due to its high content of grain protein, and the acid so formed is just as capable of producing arthritis as the acid formed from animal protein. For those who wish to continue consuming large amounts of cereal foods, it is essential to consume also large amounts of fresh fruit and raw salads which produce an alkaline effect in the body capable, at least to some degree, of neutralizing the acid.

THE COMMON COLD

Have all the world's viruses conspired lately to wipe out the human race? Or is the human race merely degenerating faster to present the viruses and germs an open invitation?

A recent report by Australian researchers (*Cecil Textbook of Medicine,* 1985, 17th edition) shows that 60% of human illness occurs in the upper respiratory tract in the form of colds, influenza and secondary bacterial infections. The survey showed an average of 5.6 infections per person per year, and 8.3 per young child.

If a person possesses an active, powerful immune system, the rate of such infections is zero. The problem is that with lipotoxemia from a bad diet, your immune system, like the rest of the body, becomes debilitated and cannot provide the protection it is designed to provide.

To illustrate this basic fact is the statement by Sir Albert Howard in his book *The Role of Insects and Fungi in Agriculture:* "For twenty one years (1910-1931) I was able to study the reaction of well-fed animals to epidemic diseases, such as rinderpest, foot-and-mouth disease, septicemia and so forth, which frequently devastated the countryside. None of my animals were segregated;

none were inoculated; they frequently came in contact with diseased stock. No case of infectious disease occurred. The reward of well-nourished protoplasm was a very high degree of disease resistance, which might even be described as immunity."

IN CONCLUSION

In the USA In 1986 just under one million people died of heart disease and 463,000 died of cancer. In the entire history of AIDS as a 'new' complaint there have been only 18,000 reported deaths from it, but unless the root of the AIDS problem is recognised, these numbers will inevitably increase.

All of these deaths resulted from errors in lifestyle, mainly errors in diet, not to mention about another half million deaths from other degenerative diseases so caused. Can you imagine two million corpses all piled up in a huge heap? Screaming headlines —

2 MILLION PEOPLE COMMIT SUICIDE

And that's only one country, one year. That's civilization today.

The great Swedish doctor Are Waerland once said: "We are not concerned wth diseases but with mistakes . . . of living. Get rid of the mistakes, and the diseases will disappear of their own accord."

There would be some excuse for the despair and death all around us if the mistakes of our civilized lifestyle were not known, but they have been known for many years and are simple to recognize and understand. In regard to cancer, at a meeting of Nobel Laureates at Lindau, Germany, June 30 1966, Dr Otto Warburg, the winner of two Nobel prizes for his discoveries of the key processes of cell respiration and various associated enzyme systems, concluded his address by saying: "Nobody today can say that one does not know what cancer and its prime cause be. On the contrary, there is no disease whose prime cause is better known; so that today ignorance is no excuse that one cannot do more about prevention. The prevention of cancer will come there is no doubt, for man wishes to survive. But how long prevention will be avoided depends on how long the prophets of agnosticism will succeed in inhibiting the application of scientific knowledge in the cancer field. In the meantime, millions of people must die of cancer unnecessarily."

These remarks of Dr Warburg's equally apply to all the other so-called diseases of civilization — asthma, arthritis, high blood pressure, failing eyesight, liver disease, kidney disease, prostate disease, tooth decay, osteoporosis, multiple sclerosis, pre-menstrual tension, migraine, constipation and so on. Like cancer, heart disease and AIDS, they are all explainable and all easily avoidable. (See *The Health Revolution*, editions three or four.)

Dr John Tilden summed it all up thus: "In chronic disease, the treatment first, last and all the time, must be with a view of getting rid of the toxemia. This consists of correcting whatever habits of life are producing enervation, and then gradually building up a normal digestion, assimilation and elimination.

"After fifty years of floundering in the great sea of medical and surgical speculation to find the causes of so-called diseases, all I could find was that all of the people were sick part of the time, a part of the people were sick all of the time — but glory be — all of the people were not sick all of the time.

"Some people get well under my treatment and friends would say I 'cured' them. Others died, and friends would say that Providence removed them. I knew I did not cure those who got well, and I did not like to acknowledge even to myself that I had killed those who died.

"It took a long time to evolve out of the one conventional idea of many diseases into the truth that there is but ONE disease, and that the four hundred catalogued so-called diseases are but different manifestations of toxemia — blood and tissue uncleanliness."

CHAPTER SEVEN

Dieting for Health

"We are not concerned with diseases but with mistakes. . .of living. Get rid of the mistakes and the diseases will disappear of their own accord."

Dr Are Waerland

The health of the body is only as good as the health, collectively, of all the body's individual cells. In turn, the health of the cells is determined by the quality of the lymph fluid that bathes them (i.e. the *milieu interieur*), which again is dependent on the purity of the bloodstream.

So while it has long been a medical dictum that 'a man is as old as his arteries', it is equally true that 'a man is as healthy as his blood'.

The composition of the blood is very complex and is maintained by the combined actions of all the vital organs. From the point of view of nutrition, it is the liver which takes in the products of digested food and re-distributes them into the bloodstream to suit the rest of the body's requirements. And it is the liver which receives back, also via the blood, the waste products of all the cells from which it sorts out what components can be used again and what must be thrown out in the urine via the kidneys. For the maintenance of correct blood sugar levels, the liver depends on information from the pancreas, a dual purpose organ which not only secretes the insulin and glucogen used in the control of blood sugar but secretes, as an entirely separate function, the primary digestive enzyme juices used in the digestion of food. In the beginning and in the end, the status of health is determined almost entirely by the quality of the diet, because it is from the materials available in the diet that the liver constructs and orchestrates the entire spectrum of chemical processes upon which life depends.

Because the Western diet contains adequate quantities of all the nutrients needed to sustain life, it is considered to be 'balanced' and capable of maintaining good health. This is true only to a point, because reasonable health can be maintained on the Western diet only as long as the digestive system, liver, and other vital organs are capable of enduring the load the diet puts upon them.

Dieting for better health then has little to do with taking vitamins, minerals and 'health foods', because when it is realized that most of the malnutrition suffered in civilization eventuates not because the diet contains deficiencies but because it contains things and combinations that are harmful, then it becomes clear that the first thing to do is to cut out the harmful things. So without making any changes in the diet at all, great improvements in health can be achieved simply by eating less, so accomplishing a purer bloodstream and at the same time getting rid of excess weight.

Although overweight is associated with increased risk of disease and shortened lifespan, it does not follow that dieting for weight loss and dieting for health are the same. Whereas proper dieting will achieve both weight adjustment and good health together, there are some slimming diets which achieve weight loss at the expense of health. Diets such as the Atkins diet, the Stillman diet and the Scarsdale diet are effective in reducing weight but are dangerous over a period. They work because they cut down (correctly) on fat and refined carbohydrate but make the mistake of substituting high protein foods as 'filler-uppers', so increasing the intake of protein from a barely tolerable level to an even less tolerable level certain to worsen toxemia and increase the risk of kidney failure and cancer.

Toxemia is the enemy, and lipotoxemia is the arch-enemy of health. The worst feature of the Western diet is all the fat in it, and therefore regardless of anything else, our first objective must be to drastically reduce the intake of fat. By virtue of unsticking the blood and improving its circulation and oxygen content, great benefits are felt within three or four days. With less impedance to the digestion by fat, putrefaction in the colon is reduced and therefore toxemia from that source is reduced too. As fat severely inhibits the function of the immune system, reduction of fat brings about vastly improved immune function, also within a few days. Regardless of which 'health diet' a person chooses, be it the European grape diet, the Pritikin diet, the Gerson diet, the Macrobiotic diet, the fruit juice diet, or just plain fasting, in all cases a great improvement in wellbeing is experienced in three or four days, the improvement being due to the fact that all these diets are low in fat.

Medical authorities, slowly getting the message, currently recommend people should reduce the amount of fat in their diet to 30%, but this is nowhere near good enough. Some benefit is felt at 20% but for proper effect the maximum should be 10%, as has already been described in previous chapters.

There are two alternative methods of reducing fat and cholesterol in the blood. Physical endurance (aerobic) exercise produces what is called the 'training effect' by which the body becomes capable of more efficiently metabolizing blood fats for the production of energy. Athletes in training therefore display lower blood viscosity, lower blood pressure, higher oxygen levels, better immune function and better general health when on the conventional Western diet than do untrained people on the same diet. The other way of coping better with high levels of dietary fat (can you guess?) is to eat the fat raw the way the primitive

Eskimos do, and allow the adipose lipase (enzyme) in the fat itself to pre-digest the fat to allow its more thorough breakdown during digestion. Not that the Western diet ever contained much whale blubber, but at least once upon a time the milk, butter and cheese was unpasteurized and contained valuable enzymes. I guess the easiest way to eliminate fat from the bloodstream is simply not to eat it in the first place, remembering that all foods contain some, the bad items being foods of animal origin, dairy products, and of course all extracted vegetable oils and anything containing them. Remember too that the body makes its own fat out of protein and carbohydrates and that when refined carbohydrates, sugar and alcohol are taken, these too will elevate the amount of fat (triglycerides) in the blood. Animal fat of course contains lots of cholesterol too, so eliminating this fat from the diet serves a double purpose.

The next step in dietary improvement of course is to reduce the amount of protein in the diet. Cutting out foods of animal origin — meat, chicken, eggs and dairy products — will achieve this because these foods are the major source of protein in the conventional diet, and by eliminating them you eliminate in one move, not only excess protein but cholesterol and excess fat as well. Conventional nutritionalists usually advise vegetarians to maintain their protein intake levels by using nuts, lentils and beans which are high in vegetable protein, but there is absolutely no need for this as our aim is to reduce protein to between five and ten per cent. On the strictest vegetarian diet it is difficult to get protein down to five per cent anyhow.

By reducing the worst ingredients of the Western diet — fat, protein, cholesterol and salt — to safe levels, you will have eliminated to a great extent the factors underlying most of the diseases of civilization, particularly atherosclerosis (heart disease), kidney disease and cancer.

Reference back to previous chapters will remind you that a lot more improvements can still be made if you are looking for the very best results, because the question comes in two parts, (a) what immediate degree of health do I want? and (b) how long do I want it to last? A moderate dietary change may restore a forty year old to good health whereas the same change may not get the desired results in a person of sixty whose vital organs are in worse condition. The forty year old, as he gets older may find he needs to be stricter with his diet to maintain good health. A lot of people claim they don't need to diet for health at all, because they have never had a day's sickness in their life. The trouble is they cannot see the degeneration going on inside them and they don't even feel it until they perhaps one day start getting chest pains or maybe feel a strange lump inside them, or spit out some blood. Thus someone, proud of their vigorous health, may suddenly overnight become a permanent invalid or even be finished for good.

It is human nature to seek pleasure and to put other things aside until forced to attend to them and for this reason most people only start thinking of their health when it starts to fail. Then they want a 'quick fix' so they can return to their indulgences again. When they find medicine is a waste of time and money they may decide to try diet. There are many diets to choose from. All of them require self discipline because to some extent or other the seductive flavors of the Western diet must be abandoned. We are addicted to these flavors and giving them up is as hard as giving up any other drug.

Temporary diets for health

In Europe the Grape diet has for years been popular in various spas and sanitoria, where sick people go to spend some weeks to recover their failing health. In a short while invalids feel great, lose weight etc. and then return home to indulge in their favorite foods again, planning on another spa holiday next year.

Other people go on fruit-juice fasts, grapefruit diets and so on and get the same wonderful results for just as long as they remain away from the Western style food. They almost always return to their old eating habits, not because they cannot break the habit but because they cannot break the addiction. Habit and addiction are not the same thing.

In the mid 1800s a wonderful health diet was invented by Dr J. H. Salisbury of New York. It was of course called the Salisbury diet and so incredibly good were the results gained by it that people travelled even from Europe to be treated by Dr Salisbury. The story of the Salisbury diet is told in a book by Dr Emmet Densmore of England called *How Nature Cures* written almost one hundred years ago. The writer was astonished to read that the diet consisted of nothing other than lean, partially cooked ground beefsteak taken three times a day preceded an hour beforehand by a pint of hot water with another pint of water taken before retiring at night. On this diet the patients all suffered a constant craving for something sweet, but all rapidly improved in health. Although potentially dangerous in the long term, the diet achieved marvellous short term results simply because it was low in fat and devoid of starch, starch being from Dr Densmore's experience the worst dietary factor of all (see chapter 10). In effect the diet was equivalent to a partial fast, and the European patients could have achieved better results and saved themselves a long trip by going to Germany and eating grapes.

Fasting

For people in well enough condition to undertake a fast this is probably the most rapid and effective way to detoxify the body and return it to full function and health. For best results the fast should continue until the body is completely detoxified and this may take anything from a week or two to several months depending on the individual case. Fasting must be carefully supervised and is outside the scope of this discussion.

Health diets for permanent adoption

The Weight Watchers' diet. This diet is calculated more to achieve weight loss than to improve health, but if followed properly both weight loss and improved health will follow. The Weight Watchers' diet could be described as 'the Western diet in moderation' and health improvement can be expected mainly as a result of eating fewer calories rather than changing the kind of food. The diet is nowhere near ideal because it still permits too much protein and fat, mayonnaise, cheese, eggs, salt and pepper. But it is better than the conventional Western diet and is a good start in the right direction.

Vegetarian diet. A true vegetarian diet permits no foods of animal origin at all. People following such a diet are known as 'vegans'. People who eat no animal flesh of any kind (or fish) but include milk, cheese and eggs in their diet are referred to as lacto-ovo-vegetarians.

The obvious advantage of vegetarianism is the absence in the diet of animal protein, animal fat and cholesterol. Lacto-ovo-vegetarians still take in these harmful substances because dairy products and eggs are high in them, and so they gain only partial benefit.

As a rule most vegetarians consume a fair amount of cereal (grain) products, lentils and beans and as a result still take in too much protein. As will be explained later, these foods are of very dubious value although they are widely accepted as 'health foods'. In addition, further harm ensues when vegetable oils are freely used, and when the vegetarian food is cooked — particularly if overcooked, salted and spiced.

Thus many vegetarians are not much better off, healthwise, than those consuming the traditional diet. However, notwithstanding these mistakes, the advantages of following the vegetarian way of life are still considerable as demonstrated by statistics on death rates quoted from the medical journal *Circulation*, Vol. 58 No. 1, July 1978. The quotation is from the text of a lecture called 'Lifestyles, Major Risk Factors, Proof and Public Policy' by noted cardiologist Dr Jeremiah Stamler.

1. "An additional comparison has recently become available, with

data on mortality, for three groups of Californian Seventh Day Adventists (non-vegetarian, lacto-ovo-vegetarian and pure vegetarian) compared with the Californian general population. Seventh Day Adventists have lower mean serum cholesterol levels than Americans generally. For 47,000 Seventh Day Adventist men aged 35 and over, age-sex-standardized, mortality rates were 34% lower for non-vegetarians, 57% lower for the lacto-ovo-vegetarians and 77% lower for the pure vegetarians compared to the general population. Seventh Day Adventists differ from the general population in other respects as well, e.g. abstinence from both alcohol and tobacco."

2. "Since the data from both animal and human studies indicate that high blood pressure and cigarette smoking are minimally significant for atherogenesis in the absence of the nutritional metabolic prerequisites, it is further reasonable and sound to designate 'rich' diet as a PRIMARY, ESSENTIAL, NECESSARY CAUSE of the current epidemic of premature atherosclerotic disease raging in the Western industrialized countries. Cigarette smoking and hypertension are important secondary or complementary causes."

The Macrobiotic diet. Any diet that drastically cuts out fat and cholesterol must, like the Salisbury diet, show good results. The Macrobiotic diet, of Japanese origin, endows great health benefits when it is adopted by people who have been on the Western diet. The diet is based on grain products, principally brown rice steamed or boiled, which accounts for over 50% of the total intake, about 25% cooked vegetables, 10% beans or lentils, 5% miso, 5% seaweed and only 5-10% raw vegetables. Fruit is not recommended and salt is allowed.

The Macrobiotic diet is claimed to be a healthy diet and indeed, by comparison to the Western diet, may appear to be so. The diet's shortcomings will be already apparent to the reader and will become even more apparent in later discussion.

The Pritikin diet. Nathan Pritikin claimed his diet to be the 'healthiest diet in the world'. If he was comparing the Pritikin diet with the traditional diets of the major population groups around the world, his claim would have been substantially correct. There is no question of the Pritikin diet's superiority over the Western diet for a start, and its emphasis on complex carbohydrates and reduction of protein and fat make it theoretically a far better diet than the traditional balanced diet espoused by today's nutritional experts.

The Pritikin diet achieves rapid, often spectacular results, first and foremost because of its very low fat content. It achieves reversal of atherosclerosis because of its low cholesterol content. It achieves reduction of blood pressure by virtue of unsticking the blood and lowering its viscosity, and by the same means permits the body's insulin to work better, so reversing diabetes. Lots of other good things happen simply because of improved circulation and more oxygen in the tissues. But the Pritikin diet too has faults which can lead to trouble if not circumvented, the main fault being that, like the Macrobiotic diet, it relies too heavily on grain products and permits too much cooking. More on this later.

The Gerson diet. Originally devised to solve the problem of migraine, the Gerson diet was found to be effective in arresting the other metabolic and degenerative diseases, and has been used with high levels of success in the treatment of cancer since the 1930s. The diet is of course very low in fat, cholesterol and protein, consisting mainly of raw vegetables, fruit and juices made from these. Some cooked vegetables and rice are permitted but the diet does not contain much grains and therefore must be considered superior to the Pritikin diet. The results demonstrated by Dr Gerson, and more lately by his daughter Charlotte, clearly demonstrate this superiority. (See chapter 8.)

The Hunza diet. The unsurpassed health and physical endurance of the legendary Hunza race was proven in exhaustive tests by Major General Sir Robert McCarrison M.D., British Army, in the 1920s to be directly attributable to the Hunza diet.

(*The Wheel of Health,* Dr G. T. Wrench, see also *The Health Revolution.*) The Hunza diet was similar to the Pritikin diet in that it contained a fair amount of wholegrain foods mainly in the form of wheatmeal bread, hardly any meat or fish, and a lot of vegetables, boiled and raw. As well, however, the diet contained liberal quantities of raw fruit, raw milk and cheese. There were no chickens, eggs, tea, sugar or rice. In the seven years he spent among the Hunzas, Dr McCarrison's medical skills were almost entirely confined to the treatment of accidental lesions, operations for granular eyelids, and the removal of senile cataracts, as other health problems were practically unknown. Dr Wrench, in his account, remarked upon the amount of raw food consumed by the Hunzas and attributed this mainly to be why they were so free of disease.

The Raw Food diet. Nobody can claim to have invented the raw food diet; it is the diet provided by Mother Nature in the first place. Dr Richard Lambe of England extolled the virtues of the raw vegetarian diet back in 1809 and described the successful use of it in the treatment of cancer patients.

Diets made up of raw fruits and/or raw vegetables have been the key to the success of the famous sanatoria in Europe, USA, Australia and elsewhere for many years. These include the Battle Creek Sanitorium started by Dr Harvey Kellogg of the USA a hundred years ago, the Bircher Benner Sanitorium in Switzerland, the Hopewood Health Centre in Australia and Dr Ann Wigmore's Hippocrates Health Centers in the USA. The advantages of eating food uncooked are many and result in health benefits unobtainable from cooked food. Some foods, such as cereals and potatoes, are difficult to digest uncooked but, as will be explained later, such foods are of dubious value anyway and are better left alone.

The Fruitarian diet. Theoretically, and in practise, a diet composed of high quality, ripe, raw fruits provides the human body with all the nutrients it needs with the very least expenditure of digestive effort, at the same time producing no toxic byproducts.

so allowing the body to detoxify itself and perform at its peak. Raw fruits are more palatable and provide more energy for a given amount than vegetables and can be prepared with less effort and less waste. Not only can the highest level of health be attained on a fruitarian diet, but because it places so much less wear and tear on the body's vital organs, degeneration is slowed down and the lifespan extended. (See chapter 12, *Dieting for Longevity.*)

The facts and fallacies of 'health foods'

When you walk into a health food store and look around, what do you see? One wall of shelves is packed with vitamins and mineral products, all expensive and all unnecessary for people on a reasonable diet. Another section displays jars of seaweed extracts, sea-salt, vegetable salts, lecithin granules and so on, all of which have dubious value. Seaweed undoubtedly contains minerals that may be light-on in some people's diets, but sea-salt, apart from the fact it contains iodine, an essential trace mineral missing from the soil in a few areas of the world, is still plain sodium chloride which is common salt — a dangerous product. Vegetable salt is a flavoring powder made from vegetable extracts but has little flavor of its own and so when you read the label on the jar it usually reveals the fact that ordinary salt or sea-salt forms part of the mixture. Lecithin extract is nearly all fat.

Then you see nuts of all kinds, dried lentils, soya beans — bins full of them — foods which contain high levels of fat and protein and are stressful to the digestive system. Shelves are stacked with bottles of vegetable oils marked 'polyunsaturated' and 'cold pressed'. These products are the most lethal 'foods' you can get.

Cookies, biscuits, energy bars, some of them high in fat and sugar, none of them as healthful as a good banana. Bins of brown rice and other grains — fair enough foods if eaten sparingly — and bins of dried fruits.

Dried fruits, if they are sun-dried and unsulfured, are good foods but very concentrated and better eaten sparingly as snacks when fresh fruit is not available.

One food item which could be considered as a health promoting food is garlic, not because it provides valuable nutrients the body needs, but because of its therapeutic medicinal property in a body handicapped by a high-fat diet. Garlic, onions and other herbal extracts such as vitamin E, have the effect of unsticking the blood to permit improved circulation. Used for this purpose these products are more medicines than foods, but at least garlic tastes good.

The contents of health food stores can be considered health-giving only to the extent they are less harmful than meat, chicken and dairy products. The only foods that qualify to be called health foods, using the true meaning of the word 'health', are fresh fruits and vegetables; you can maintain good health indefinitely on these but the same cannot be said for the general run of foods available in health food stores.

Summarizing health diets

The single common denominator possessed by all effective health diets is the drastic lowering of the fat content, which allows the blood-stream to clear itself of fat and allows the red blood cells and blood platelets to unstick, so reducing the blood viscosity and permitting its free circulation and oxygen-carrying ability. The enormous improvement in wellbeing that results from this single factor of improved blood condition has nothing to do with anything contained in the diet — the benefit stems from what has been taken out of the diet.

So great is the improvement of health and wellbeing achieved by the simple expedient of improving the circulation that the beneficiaries think they have struck the jackpot; they think they have discovered the perfect diet, be it the Grape diet, the Macrobiotic diet, the Pritikin diet, the Gerson diet or maybe even the Salisbury diet. And this is easy to understand, but there is more to good health than just improving the blood circulation. What about the delicate chemistry of the blood? What about the avoidance of toxemia? The wear and tear on our internal organs? The wastage of digestive energy and valuable enzymes?

Insidious degeneration can continue undetected in a body apparently brimming with vigorous health. Probably the best example of this is the constant occurrence of sudden death by heart attack of extremely fit athletes and runners. Right up until their sudden collapse, which usually occurs during or just after vigorous activity, these people display all the signs of good health. Their blood viscosity is low because they can metabolize fat quickly from their blood and so their blood pressure is good, they feel good because their blood contains plenty of oxygen, they don't 'catch' colds because their immune systems are performing properly. They are healthy in this sense, but when death overtakes them autopsies reveal coronary arteries blocked with cholesterol. They had been under the illusion that endurance exercise prevents heart disease; but the evidence is now clear that physical training does not prevent the accumulation of dietary cholesterol in the arteries, it merely maintains a better blood flow and prevents the usual symptoms of heart disease from being displayed.

Nathan Pritikin was the first one to loudly warn the public of the dangerous illusion that athletes could indulge in a high cholesterol diet and get away with it. But there are other illusions of which Pritikin was not aware. Avoiding heart disease is not the be-all and end-all in the quest for good health.

Clean arteries and thin blood are the prime essentials and these are easily accomplished on the Pritikin diet providing the diet is properly followed. The next step is attending to the actual chemistry of the blood and how perfect chemistry can be achieved with the least wear and tear on the vital organs. This involves further investigation into nutrition and the enzymes that make improved nutrition possible. The subject becomes a little different from that of dieting for immediate health benefits, it becomes one of gaining long-term benefits, the subject of chapter 12 — *Dieting for Longevity.*

CHAPTER EIGHT

Doctor Max Gerson

"He was a medical genius who walked among us."
Dr Albert Schweitzer

Doctors are human, they follow their training and plod through life like other people, some with enquiring minds and some with blinkers on. As each generation of doctors gains experience many of them question the value of medicine because the results they observe are so dismal. Granted, most of their day-to-day patients survive, but usually not because of medicine, but despite it.

You would think when even little children know that some things are 'good for you' and other things are 'bad for you', that doctors, having once been children themselves, when confronted by a very sick patient, would instantly enquire, "Have you been eating anything bad for you?"

But they don't, as a rule, because their training has totally misorientated their minds away from Nature and the fact that in Nature health is the universal state. Like most civilized people, doctors accept disease as simply a fairly normal part of life. But not everybody, not all doctors.

There have always been, through the generations, doctors with enquiring minds, doctors who when disappointed with the status quo, look for something better. Doctors like Thomas Sydenham, William Harvey, Richard Lambe, Russell Trall, Louis Kuhne, Charles De Lacy Evans, Emmet Densmore, Robert Bell, Robert McCarrison, John Tilden, Edward Howell, William Koch, Cornelius Moerman, Arbuthnot Lane, Ferdinand Sauerbruch, Robert Mendelsohn, to name a few. There are many names, but unfortunately, not enough of them. Max Gerson was one of this breed.

Max Gerson graduated in medicine in Germany in 1909. He practised conventional medicine but himself was plagued with migraine and could do nothing to get rid of it. That is until he started experimenting with diet. Eventually he developed a diet low in salt, protein and fat, upon which his migraine headaches no longer occurred, and so of course from that time on he treated all his migraine patients by putting them on his low salt, low protein, low fat diet, whereupon they too became free of headaches.

That this diet could allow the body to heal itself from other disease conditions was at first not apparent to Dr Gerson, but eventually this realization occurred to him in rather a dramatic way. The description of this important incident is described in New York writer S. J. Haught's book *Has Doctor Max Gerson a True Cancer Cure?** (1962) as follows:

> When the young doctor at first began to use his new therapy on his migraine patients he was jubilant to observe them all respond the same as he had done himself. But even more spectacular was his discovery when a migraine patient, whose job was in jeopardy due to his repeated absences, begged him for help. Dr Gerson noticed the man's eyelids, cheek and nose were being eaten away by disease — *lupus vulgaris*, tuberculosis of the skin. Nothing, he thought, could be done for that — lupus was an incurable disease — so he prescribed his diet for migraine and sent the patient home.
>
> Not long afterwards the patient returned. "And how is the migraine?" the doctor asked.
>
> "Gone, all gone!" happily exclaimed the man, "I haven't missed a day's work since!" He couldn't control his excitement. "Doctor, do you notice anything else? My face?"
>
> Dr Gerson leaned closer. Was it possible — the same man?
>
> "Yes, it's true," said the patient. "My lupus — that horrible, ugly lupus — vanished! Like a miracle!"
>
> It was hard to say who was the more elated — doctor or patient. Would the old disfiguring scourge of lupus also respond to the

*Reprinted with the title *Cancer, Think Curable* published by The Gerson Institute, Bonita, California.

migraine diet?

Before long, lupus patients were flocking to Dr Gerson's door, clamoring for the miracle they'd heard about. And wonder of wonders, the blessing repeated itself.

Other doctors, who had been echoing the ageless shibboleth of organized medicine, "Nothing can be done," were infuriated with Dr Gerson's success. They brought charges against him for treating skin diseases, which was not his specialty.

"I'll be very proud to be punished for curing lupus," Dr Gerson told them.

He continued to cure lupus, and by 1928 he had compiled his findings. Newspapers and magazines throughout Europe hailed the discovery, and offers from many countries descended upon the young doctor.

The bitterness of the medical fraternity knew no bounds. "It is not scientific!" they cried.

"My answer is very short," was Dr Gerson's reply. "If it is not scientific to cure the incurable, then I am not scientific!"

By this time Gerson had devoted many years to his research. What a pity he had never heard of Dr Richard Lambe who in England had gone through all this one hundred years before. It is of interest to note also that Dr Louis Kuhne had employed similar dietary means to achieve exactly the same results at his clinic in Leipzig, Germany only thirty years beforehand. I wonder if Dr Gerson had ever read Kuhne's book *The New Science of Healing*?

Lupus vulgaris is not a very pleasant sight and for that matter, not a very pleasant topic, except when you can relate of the happiness of people cured of this 'incurable' disease.* But to illustrate further the peculiar social behavior of humans and how they unwittingly bring so much trouble upon themselves, here is a further story about lupus from Germany, taken from the autobiography of Dr Ferdinand Sauerbruch,** the master surgeon who pioneered thoracic surgery and was the first to operate successfully on the human heart. Dr Sauerbruch relates:

*Lupus is today still considered by most doctors to be incurable.

**Author of *A Surgeon's Life*, 1953. (Also published under the title of *Master Surgeon.*)

"I was sitting in a train traveling from Munich to Davos, where I had once again been invited. It had been an exhausting day and I tried to sleep, but in vain. I had probably drunk too much coffee. Grimly I leaned back and tried to read the medical journals I had with me. After we had crossed into Switzerland, another traveler got into my compartment. The man seemed bored, and it was plain that he was looking for a chance to open conversation. He irritated me by shuffling his feet, twitching his legs, fidgeting with his clothes, and by his general restlessness. Before long, he made his opening move.

"Are you going to Davos, too?"

"Yes," I growled.

After a very short silence, he tried again. "Are you a patient?"

"No."

He peered across to try and read the titles of the periodicals which I had thrown down beside me on the seat.

"So you are a doctor going to Davos?"

"No, I am not."

"Thank God for that. Doctors are fools. All but one."

We rattled on through the night. I was desperately tired. I could not read, my eyes were aching, yet in spite of myself I was curious concerning this exception. It was not difficult to set him off again. As I stared at him, he asked, "What can you see on my face?"

"Burns," I suggested.

"Burns!" he cried. "These aren't burns. They are the scars of skin tuberculosis, and I was cured of it by this doctor."

"What!" I exclaimed, though with some restraint. Skin tuberculosis, lupus, an unsightly disease for which there was no known cure. I decided that my fellow traveler was just bragging. "There's no cure for lupus."

"There used to be no cure," he replied. "But one has been found. I have been cured."

Before he realized what was happening, I was unfastening his jacket and shirt, for we were alone in the compartment and some distance from the next station. And on his chest I saw large areas of perfectly healed lupus. I asked him to tell me his story. From his accent, I judged him to be Russian.

The disease, he said, had developed in his home country; he had gone from doctor to doctor. Being well-to-do, he had been able to afford treatment abroad and had visited German hospitals — in vain. Feeling more and more like a medieval leper, he had been on the brink of suicide, when he was told that there was a doctor named Gerson in Bielefeld who claimed to be able to cure lupus. He decided to go to him. Why not? The effects of the disease on his face were such that he would soon be forced to retire from the world. People shrank from him, and few hotels would admit him.

As soon as Dr Gerson saw him, he exclaimed, "Ha! Lupus, lupus vulgaris."

"Can you help me?"

"Of course I can help you." And he did.

I asked him how he had done so.

"By diet."

In the whole range of medical literature, there was no reference to the treatment of lupus by diet.

"When I was cured," he continued. "I went to all the famous doctors who had told me there was no cure, and they all laughed at me. Doctors!"

"Did you ever go to Sauerbruch?" I asked.

"It wouldn't have been any use. He's in Munich, and anyway, he always quarrels with everybody, shouts and bellows at them. He wouldn't listen."

I told him that I knew Sauerbruch and that I could guarantee that Sauerbruch would see him. And then he told me why he was going to Switzerland. He was hoping to acquire a building for the treatment of lupus patients free-of-charge. It was to be a gesture of gratitude for his release from this dreaded scourge. But he knew that he would need the support of some prominent man, for Dr Gerson's name was practically unknown.

"Do not forget to call on Sauerbruch," were my parting words to him. "I shall see that you are received by him."

About a fortnight later, the Russian was shown into my office, accompanied by a modest man with a highly intelligent face. Dr Gerson himself, I guessed.

"So you are Sauerbruch yourself!"

Gerson declared that he had cured a number of patients by excluding salt from their diet entirely. My Russian visitor was one of them. And of his cure there could be no doubt, however amazing his claim might seem. I could see no apparent connection between treatment and cure, but that did not prevent me from beginning a series of experiments immediately.

I put my assistant, Dr Hermannsdorfer, in charge of a wing of the clinic which was fitted up as a lupus station. The patients were to be fed in accordance with Dr Gerson's diet. Lupus patients were found. We securely barred doors and windows to prevent escape. A person who, over a long period, is given food with no salt at all suffers from his situation.

Dr Gerson returned to his practice and I promised to keep him informed of our progress. Results were catastrophic. We kept the patients locked up for weeks. Not a grain of salt went into their food, but there was no trace of improvement. On the contrary, in each case, the disease advanced according to rule. Dr Hermannsdorfer and I were at a loss, thinking of the Russian who had been cured, and of humble Dr Gerson in whom we had put complete faith.

We felt we must drop the experiment. Sadly I wrote to Dr Gerson, telling him of the failure of the experiment and our decision to close the lupus ward. I dictated that letter in the morning. That afternoon, a sister called me to an emergency case: a patient had a severe post-operative hemorrhage. I hastened along corridors and down stairs and did what was necessary. Pensively I was strolling back along the corridor near the lupus ward, when I saw a nurse, the fattest nurse in the building, carrying an enormous tray loaded with sausages, bowls of cream, and jugs of beer. It was four o'clock in the afternoon, hardly the time for such a feast in a hospital. In amazement, I stopped and asked her where on earth she was going with all that food. And then the whole story came out.

"I couldn't bear it any longer, Herr Geheimrat," she explained. "Those poor patients with skin T.B. The stuff they are given — no one could eat it."

She was astonished when I dashed her tray to the ground. It was one of the occasions when I completely lost my temper. Every day, at four o'clock when no one was around, she had been taking the patients a nice, appetizing, well-seasoned meal.

I sent off a telegram to Dr Gerson, asking him not to open the letter I had written him. We were back at the beginning again, and from that moment we took extra precautions in guarding the lupus wing. In comparison, a prison would have been a holiday camp. Soon, Dr Gerson was proved right. Nearly all our patients recovered; their sores almost disappeared under our very eyes. In this experiment involving 450 patients, only four could not be cured by Dr Gerson's saltless diet."

Now at this time surgeons were regarded as the heroes of medicine and Dr Sauerbruch was the leading surgeon of Germany, famous in world medical circles, and who moved among the ranks of royalty and statesmen. Dr Gerson, with his now-proven track record and supported by Dr Sauerbruch, suddenly became not only 'respectable' in German medical circles but at the same time, a leading figure.

In 1933, he was scheduled to address the Berlin Medical Association and demonstrate his cured 'incurables' (his first successes with cancer were achieved in 1928). His address was set down for May 5, 1933.

People blame Adolf Hitler and his Nazi regime for the destruction and deaths of millions of people during the days of World War II. But there were other tragedies of that Nazi era, perhaps the greatest being that Dr Gerson's concepts were denied to a world ready to receive them.

In early 1933 political upheaval occurred in Germany and Hitler and his Nazi Party took over. Max Gerson was a Jew, and in March he was forced to flee with his family to Vienna for the safety of their lives. He remained in Vienna until forced again to flee — to Paris, and then to New York, where he arrived in 1938.

In New York Dr Gerson had to start all over again. He attended school with little children in order to learn English, and at the age of 57 he had to sit for all the American medical exams to gain his license to practise medicine again.

With the advent of WWII there was strong anti-German feeling in the USA, and strong opposition from the American Medical Association to unorthodox medical practice, and to really make things hard, Dr Gerson chose cancer as his specialty. The hardest part of all was that the majority of his patients were terminal cases, given up as hopeless by the best cancer specialists in the USA. Meanwhile, back in Germany, Dr Gerson's entire family of seven brothers and sisters had been murdered in concentration camps.

Nevertheless, despite the handicaps under which he worked and despite the fact that his patients were considered by other doctors to be as good as dead, this unflagging medical genius was able to prove a 50% recovery rate in the ranks of his cancer patients, and a success rate of almost 100% with other degenerative diseases.

In 1946 Dr Gerson became the first physician to demonstrate recovered cancer patients before a US Congressional committee. This Senate Committee was holding hearings on a bill to find means of curing and preventing cancer. Unfortunately the medical lobby supporting the orthodox treatment of cancer by surgery, radiation and chemotherapy caused the defeat by four votes of the Senate Bill which could have supported extensive research into the Gerson therapy.

Whether motivated by professional jealousy, fear of the unknown, fear of bankruptcy or plain stupidity, the American Medical Association knowingly suppressed Max Gerson's work equally as well as Adolf Hitler and his Nazis had done unknowingly.

Worn out, Dr Gerson died in 1959, of pneumonia, aged 78, just after the publication of his final work, the book *A Cancer Therapy — Results of Fifty Cases,* a book which should be on every doctor's desk and be compulsory reading for all medical students.

Dr Gerson, during his fifty years of constant medical practise, was the author of fifty five published scientific works and of course many others that were refused publication in orthodox journals.

Charitably, in the preface to his book, Dr Gerson concludes:

"The history of medicine reveals that reformers who bring new ideas into the general thinking and practice of physicians have a difficult time. Very few physicians like to change their medical approaches. The majority practise what they have learned and apply the treatments of the text-books more or less automatically. Right from the beginning, the physician wants most of all to help the patient. He hesitates to take risks for his patients by applying a non-recognized treatment. The history of science, art and technique shows that each new idea has been fought bitterly; most of the reformers did not live to see the realization of their ideas.

"This is one of the reasons why developments in culture made very slow progress all through the centuries; they were restrained forcefully.

"I was in a more favorable position. Ninety to ninety five per cent of my patients were far advanced (terminal) cases without any risk to take; either all recognized treatments had failed or the patients were inoperable from the beginning. It takes some time to acquire enough experience to see progress, results, or failures."

The great Dr Albert Schweitzer, concert organist, humanitarian and physician, the recipient of two Nobel Prizes, was himself freed of diabetes under Dr Gerson's care and his wife 'cured' of tuberculosis in the days when these diseases were considered incurable and fatal.

After Dr Gerson's death Dr Schweitzer said of him: "I see in him one of the most eminent geniuses in the history of medicine. He possessed something elemental. Out of the deepest thought about the nature of disease and the process of healing, he came to walk along new paths with great success. He leaves a legacy which commands attention and which will assure him his due place."

***Translation of the Titles of Scientific Works by Max Gerson, M.D.**

1907 Dissertation Article: Influence of the Artificial Hyperemia and Blood Transfusions in the Treatment of Fractures in the Hip Joint.

1910 Bromocol Poisoning. Aerztliche Sachverstaendigen-Zeitung.

1916 Myasthenic Bulbar Paralysis — Berliner Klinische Wochenschr. No. 51.

1918 Reflex Hyperesthesia. Zeitschrift fuer die gesamte Neurologie und Psychiatrie.

1919 Paralysis Found in Diphtheria Carriers. Berliner Klinische Wochenschrift, No. 12.

1921 Concerning the Etiology of Multiple Sclerosis. Deutsche Zeitschrift fuer Nervenheilkunde.

1924 Constitutional Basis for Nervous Symptoms. Fortschritte der Medizin, No. 1. P. 9.

1926 Experiments Attempting to Influence Severe Forms of Tuberculosis Through Dietetic Treatment. Muenchener Medizinische Wochenschrift, No. 2 and 3.

1929 Origin and Development of the Dietetic Treatment of Tuberculosis. Die Medizinische Welt 1929, No. 37.

1929 Treatment of Rickets and Tuberculosis. Deutsche Medizinische Wochenschrift 1929. No. 38.

1930 Several Experiments with the Gerson Diet in Tuberculosis. Medizinische Welt 1930.

1930 Salt Association with Migraine (an early factor in dietetic treatment). Verhandlungen der Deutschen Gesellschaft fuer Innere Medizin 1930. P.129, No. 23.

1930 Basic Approaches to the Gerson Diet. Muenchener Medizinische Wochenschrift No. 23. P.967.

1930 Phosphorus, Cod Liver Oil and the Gerson Diet in the Treatment of Tuberculosis. Deutsche Medizinische Wochenschrift No. 12.

1930 Several Factors in Dietetic Treatment of Pulmonary Tuberculosis. Zeitschrift fuer Aerztliche Fortbildung. No. 11.

1931 Nicotine as a Deterrent Factor in the Treatment of Lupus. Verhandlungen der Deutschen Gesellschaft Fuer Innere Medizin.

1931 Several Experiments in the Dietary Treatment of Tuberculosis. Verhandlungen der Deutschen Gesellschaft fuer Innere Medizin.

1931 Resume of Varying Sensory Factors in the Treatment of Lupus. Verhandlungen der Deutschen Gesellschaft fuer Innere Medizin.

1931 Basis Underlying Discontinuance of Salt Free Diet in Tuberculosis Sanitariums. Deutsche Medizinische Wochenschrift, 1931. No. 8.

1931 The Dietetic Problems of the Present Day in the Treatment of Tuberculosis. The Journal of State Medicine Vol. XXXLX No. 8, London.

1931 Sedimentation in the Dietetic Treatment of Lung Tuberculosis. Zeitschrift fuer Tuberculose 1932. Bd. 63 Heft 5.

1932 The Gerson Diet in Chronic Pulmonary Spastic Diseases and Hypertension. Wiener Klinische Wochenschrift 1932. No. 13.

1932 Observations on the Gerson Diet. Wiener Klinische Wochenschrift No. 37. 1932.

1932 The Gerson Diet in Practice — Technisch — Pharmazeutische Aerztezeitung. Wein 1932. No. 20.

1932 Dietary Treatment of Migraine and Pulmonary Tuberculosis. Wiener Klinische Wochenschrift 1932. No. 24.

1932 Gerson Diet on Pulmonary Tuberculosis and Migraine. Mitteilungen des Volksgesundheitsamtes. Jahrgang 1932. Wien, Heft 9.

1934 Psychic Reactions During the Gerson Diet in Pulmonary Tuberculosis. Psychotherapeutische Praxis. Vol. 1, Heft 4,

1934.

1935 High Fluid and Potassium Diet as Treatment in Cardiorenal Insufficiene. Muenchener Medizinische Wochenschrift No. 15.

1935 Feeding of the Tubercular. Wiener Klinische Wochenschrift No. 9.

1935 Non-Specific Desensitations by Means of Diet in Allergic Skin Diseases. Dermatologische Wochenschrift 1935. No. 15.

1935 The Recession of Inflammation in Gerson Diet with Special Reference to Tubercular Inflammations. Wiener Klinische Wochenschrift 1935. No. 25.

1935 The Administration of Liver Extract in Relation to Diet in the Treatment of Chronic Diseases. Wiener Medizinische Wochenschrift 1935. No. 40.

1935 The Gerson Diet in Home Practice. Der Oesterreichische Arzt. Folge 2, Jahrgang 2.

1941 Feeding the German Army. New York State Journal of Medicine. 1471. 41 1941.

1943 Some Aspects of the Problem of Fatigue. The Medical Record, New York. June 1943.

1945 Dietary Considerations in Malignant Neoplastic Disease. Review of Gastroenterology. Vol. 12, No. 6, Pages 419 to 425. Nov.-Dec. 1945.

1948 The Significance of the Content of Soil to Human Disease.

1949 Effect of a Combined Dietary Regime on Patients with Malignant Tumors. Experimental Medicine and Surgery. New York, Vol. VII, Nov. 4, 1949.

1954 No Cancer in Normal Metabolism. Medizinische Klinik, Munich. Jan.29, 1954, No. 5, page 175-179.

1954 Cancer a Problem of Metabolism. Medizinische Klinik, Munich. No. 26, June 25, 1954.

1955 Cancer is a Problem of Soil, Nutrition, Metabolism.

1955 Are Soil, Food and Metabolic Disturbances Basically

Responsible for Cancer Development?

1955 The Gerson Therapy and Practice in the Prevention of and Treatment for Cancer.

1955 Five Case Histories.

1956 Cancer Development and Treatment. Lecture at the Academy of Applied Nutrition (Pasadena).

1956 Rehabilitation of the Cancer Patient.

1956 The Problem of Cancer Based upon the Law of Totality.

1956 The Historic Development of the Combined Dietary Regime in Cancer.

1957 Can Cancer be Prevented? Prevention Magazine.

1957 New Therapeutical Approach to Cancer.

1957 Cancer — Reflected Symptoms of Abnormal Metabolism.

Books

1930 My Diet. Edited — Berlin 1930.

1934 Therapy of Lung Tuberculosis. Franz Deuticke, Wien — Leipzig 1934 (with monographs and X-ray pictures of the cases).

1954 Diet Therapy in Malignant Diseases (Cancer). Scala, Handbuch der Dietik, Wien, Franz Deuticke, 1954.

1958 A Cancer Therapy — Results of Fifty Cases. Totality Books.

CHAPTER NINE

Modern Medicine — A Snare and a Delusion

Is it not possible that modern humanistic man, excited by the success of the scientific method, and exalted by his liberation from the absurdities of medieval thought, has been carried away into a new period of dogmatic folly only a little less absurd than that which preceded it? Could he be making a gigantic mistake?
Alister Hardy — *The Spiritual Nature of Man*

It has been reported that from the ranks of doctors come the highest rates of suicides and drug dependency of all the occupations in society. Does this mean that doctors are more likely than others to become disillusioned and unhappy, that the career which once promised so much satisfaction at the start turns sour when the promise is not fulfilled? How many doctors, after working so hard to gain their qualifications, come to realize they have become little more than licensed drug pushers for the international drug cartels?

Many such doctors have reacted positively to set things right but usually they are considered eccentrics who are out to spoil a good set-up, and their complaints are ignored. Rejected and derided by their peers, a lot of them write books to get their message out of the barricade surrounding the medical profession, direct to the public. As books like these are written with great dedication and are based on direct observations made through the course of long medical careers, they make the best reading a medical student could get, but of course none are to be found in medical libraries anywhere.

A hundred years ago Dr Emmet Densmore and his wife, also a medical doctor, collaborated to write a book called *How Nature Cures*. In this book the fallacies surrounding orthodox medicine were exposed, and to support his opinions Dr Densmore quoted some of the prominent physicians of the time who, like the Densmores, had awakened to the fact that orthodox medicine for the treatment of common diseases was a waste of effort bordering on the farcical. A few of the quotations were:

Professor Alonzo Clark, New York College of Physicians and Surgeons: "In their zeal to do good, physicians have done much harm. They have hurried thousands to the grave who would have recovered if left to Nature."

John Mason Good, MD, FRS: "The efforts of medicine on the human system are in the highest degree uncertain, except indeed, that they have destroyed more lives than war, pestilence and famine combined."

Dr Eliphalet Kimball: "There is doctorcraft as well as priestcraft . . . Physicians have slain more than war. An instrument of death in their hands, bleeding, calomel, and other medicines have done more than powder and ball. The public would be infinitely better off without professed physicians. In weak constitutions Nature can be assisted. Good nursing is necessary, and sometimes roots and herbs do good. In strong constitutions medicine is seldom needed in sickness. To a man with a good constitution, and guided by reason in his course of living, sickness would be impossible."

Sir John Forbes: "Some patients get well with the aid of medicines, some without, and still more in spite of it."

Oliver Wendell Holmes, author and Professor of Anatomy, Harvard University: "The disgrace of medicine has been that colossal system of self deception, in obedience to which mines have been emptied of their cankering minerals, the entrails of animals taken for their impurities, the poison bag of reptiles drained for their venom, and all the inconceivable absurdities thus obtained thrust down the throats of human beings suffering simply of some want of organization, nourishment or vital stimulation.

"If all the drugs were cast into the sea, it would be so much better for man, and so much the worse for the fishes."

There were a great many other such quotations, the most descriptive of the situation being the one from the great physician and physiologist Professor Francois Magendie, President of the French Academy of Science: "Let us no longer wonder at the lamentable want of success which marks our practise, when there is scarcely a sound physiological principle among us. I hesitate not to declare, no matter how sorely I should wound our vanity, that so gross is our ignorance of the real nature of the physiological disorder called disease, that it would perhaps be better to do nothing, and resign the complaint into the hands of Nature, than to act as we are frequently compelled to do, without knowing the why and wherefore of our conduct, at the obvious risk of hastening the end of the patient.

"Gentlemen, medicine is a great humbug. I know it is called a science. Science indeed! It is nothing like science. Doctors are merely empirics when they are not charlatans. We are as ignorant as men can be. Who knows anything in the world about medicine? Gentlemen, you have done me a great honor to come here to attend my lectures, and I must tell you frankly now, in the beginning, that I know nothing in the world about medicine, and I don't know anybody who does know anything about it . . .I repeat, nobody knows anything about medicine . . .

"We are collecting facts in the right spirit, and I dare say, in a century or so, the accumulation of facts may enable our successors to form a medical science. Who can tell me how to cure the headache, or the gout, or disease of the heart? Nobody. Oh, you tell me the doctors cure people. I grant you people are cured, but how are they cured? Gentlemen, Nature does a great deal, imagination a great deal; doctors — devilishly little when they don't do any harm."

Frank statements, made a hundred years ago. Since then it is claimed, medicine has indeed become a science — or has it? If Doctor Magendie were alive today and were to enquire "Who can tell me how to cure the headache, or the gout, or the disease of the heart?" he would be forced again to conclude — nobody. Doctors can drug the symptoms of headache, gout, heart disease and most other complaints, but the patients are not cured, and many of them die prematurely as a result of the drugs.

The fact of the matter is there is not, and cannot ever be, such a thing as a medical 'cure' for anything. Only Nature can heal, but in their ignorance of this fact doctors still continue to hopefully pour into their patients the drugs recommended to them by the real controllers of the big medical show, the drug companies.

In 1973, doctors in Israel went on strike and reduced their total daily patient contacts from 65,000 to only 7000. The strike lasted a month and during that time the death-rate, according to the Jerusalem Burial Society, dropped 50%. In 1976 in Bogota, Columbia, doctors for a period of 52 days refused to treat all except emergency cases, and in that time the death-rate fell by 35%. In the same year, during a 'slow-down' by doctors in Los Angeles, the death-rate there dropped 18%. Obviously, Dr Densmore's opinions are still valid today.

Headaches, gout, heart disease, cancer, hypertension, diabetes, arthritis, MS, osteoporosis, premenstrual tension, asthma, the common cold, herpes, AIDS — the list goes on — all incurable still — regardless of the claims and promises of 'medical science'. Transplanting hearts, kidneys and livers cannot be called curing;

pumping insulin into diabetics who are diabetic only because of their high-protein, high-fat diet, is not a cure either, nor is cutting out a tumor and hoping like hell another will not take its place. Despite 20th century technology and the admirable advances in lifesaving surgery and 'crisis' medicine, for the most part modern medicine has advanced hardly at all in the last one hundred years, in regard to solving the problem of common diseases. In fact there are more common diseases today than ever there were, and the list is growing.

Medicine is in a rut pointing the wrong way. The medical profession, like any other profession, is comprised of only a few outstanding individuals out of a great multitude, all doing the best they can according to the way they have been trained. For some doctors medicine is a labor of love, to others it is merely a lucrative and prestigious career. One way or another, in the status quo of society, doctors have secured a highly favored niche, and like others so favored, are not likely to welcome any form of change. Thus medicine is an extremely conservative profession, and not being answerable to higher authority, can cover-up its shortcomings and run as a protected monopoly, virtually a law unto itself.

Doctors, over the past hundred years, despite their constant failures, have contrived to create the impression their services are of indispensable value; they have become so highly organized and influential that they have further contrived government legislation which protects them from competition under the pretext that they are protecting the public from charlatans. These achievements have been gained by the various medical associations which are the most powerful unions in the world and which, knowingly or unknowingly, have allowed the practise of medicine to become the drug-orientated pawn of the drug companies.

Mesmerised by the continuous flow of propaganda from the multi-billion dollar drug companies, the ordinary hard-working doctor, knowing almost nothing about the etiology of disease, has become an innocent drug-pusher in danger of getting writer's cramp from scribbling out prescriptions.

To what extent the average doctor realizes how farcical the situation really is in relation to treating disease, would be difficult to ascertain, but one way or another the public deception is maintained. Medicine men, both primitive and modern, maintain with varying degrees of success, an air of competence and mystique which sets them apart from ordinary people and disguises the fact they are quite ordinary people too, with human shortcomings and inner doubts. How is this gigantic deception maintained? It is maintained mainly by virtue of the fact that the healing power of Nature is so powerful. People actually recover in most cases in spite of the medical treatment they receive, and the chronically sick struggle to stay alive despite the drugs pumped into them. The illusion is that whatever good has eventuated has been achieved by the medicine, and of course when someone in pain is relieved of the pain by medicine at least some credit must be paid to drugs even if their side-effects are damaging. But as Dr Ronald Glasser says in his book *The Body is the Hero*, the real healing is achieved by the body itself, while the doctor gets the credit.

Books like Dr Glasser's put the true perspective on modern medicine. There are many others on the topic that would put the fear of death in you, perhaps the most informative one on the subject being *Confessions of a Medical Heretic* by Dr Robert S. Mendelsohn of Chicago (1979).

Dr Mendelsohn has been in medical practise for over thirty five years; he was Chairman of the Medical Licensing Committee of the State of Illinois and the recipient of numerous awards for excellence in medicine and medical instruction. He is currently the Associate Professor of Preventive Medicine at the University of Illinois, and in the introduction to his book he has this to say:

"I do not believe in Modern Medicine. I am a medical heretic.

My aim in this book is to persuade you to become a heretic, too.

I haven't always been a medical heretic. I once believed in Modern Medicine.

In medical school, I failed to look deeply into a study that was going on around me, of the effects of the hormone DES — because I believed. Who could have suspected that twenty years later we would discover that DES causes vaginal cancer and genital abnormalities in children born to women receiving the drug during pregnancy?

I confess that I failed to be suspicious of oxygen therapy for premature infants, even though the best equipped and most advanced premature nurseries had an incidence of partial or total blindness of around ninety per cent of all low birth weight infants. A few miles away, in a large, less 'advanced' hospital, the incidence of this condition — retrolental fibroplasia — was less than ten per cent. I asked my professors in medical school to explain the difference. And I believed them when they said the doctors in the poorer hospital just didn't know how to make the correct diagnosis.

A year or two later it was proved that the cause of retrolental fibroplasia was the high concentrations of oxygen administered to the premies. The affluent medical centers had higher rates of blinding simply because they could afford the very best nursery equipment: the most expensive and modern plastic incubators which guaranteed that all the oxygen pumped in reached the infant. At the poorer nurseries, however, old-fashioned incubators were used. They looked like bathtubs with very loose metal lids. They were so leaky that it made very little difference how much oxygen was pumped in: not enough reached the infant to blind it.

I still believed when I took part in a scientic paper on the use of the antibiotic Terramycin in treating respiratory conditions in premature babies. We claimed there were no side effects. Of course there weren't. We didn't wait long enough to find out that not only didn't Terramycin — or any other antibiotic — do much good for these infections, but that it — and other tetracycline antibiotics — left thousands of children with yellow-green teeth and tetracycline deposits in their bones.

And I confess that I believed in the irradiation of tonsils, lymph nodes, and the thymus gland. I believed my professors when they said that of course radiation was dangerous, but that the doses we were using were absolutely harmless.

Years later — around the time we found out that the 'absolutely harmless' radiation sown a decade or two before was now reaping a harvest of thyroid tumors — I couldn't help wondering when some of my former patients came back with nodules of their thyroids: Why are you coming back to me? To *me*, who did this to you in the first place?

But I no longer believe in Modern Medicine.

I believe that despite all the super technology and elite bedside manner that's supposed to make you feel about as well cared for as an astronaut on the way to the moon, the greatest danger to your health is the doctor who practices Modern Medicine.

I believe that Modern Medicine's treatments for disease are seldom effective, and that they're often more dangerous than the diseases they're designed to treat.

I believe the dangers are compounded by the widespread use of dangerous procedures for non-diseases.

I believe that more than ninety per cent of Modern Medicine could disappear from the face of the earth — doctors, hospitals, drugs and equipment — and the effect on our health would be immediate and beneficial.

I believe that Modern Medicine has gone too far, by using in everyday situations extreme treatments designed for critical conditions.

Every minute of every day Modern Medicine goes too far, because Modern Medicine *prides itself* on going too far. A recent article, 'Cleveland's Marvelous Medical Factory', boasted of the Cleveland Clinic's 'accomplishments' last year: 2,980 open-heart operations, 1.3 million laboratory tests, 73,320 electrocardiograms, 7,770 full-body x-ray scans, 210,378 other radiologic studies, 24,368 surgical procedures.'

Not one of these procedures has been proved to have the least little bit to do with maintaining or restoring health. And the article, which was published in the Cleveland Clinic's own magazine, fails to boast or even mention that any people were helped by any of this expensive extravagance. That's because the product of this factory is not health at all.

So when you go to the doctor, you're seen not as a person who needs help with his or her health, but as a potential market for the medical factory's products.

If you're pregnant, you go to the doctor and he treats you as if you're sick. Childbirth is a nine-month disease which must be treated, so you're sold on intravenous fluid bags, fetal monitors, a host of drugs, the totally unnecessary episiotomy, and — the top of the line product — the Caesarean delivery!

If you make the mistake of going to the doctor with a cold or the flu, he's liable to give you antibiotics, which are not only powerless against colds and flu but which leave you more likely to come down with worse problems.

If your child is a little too peppy for his teacher to handle, your doctor may go too far and turn him into a drug dependent.

If your new baby goes off his or her feed for a day and doesn't gain weight as fast as the doctor's manual says, he might barrage your breastfeeding with drugs to halt the natural process and make room in the baby's tummy for man-made formula, which is dangerous.

If you're foolish enough to make that yearly visit for a routine examination, the receptionist's petulance, the other patients' cigarette smoke, or the doctor's very presence could raise your blood pressure enough so that you won't go home empty-handed. Another life 'saved' by antihypertensive drugs. Another sex life down the drain, since more impotence is caused by drug therapy than by psychological problems.

If you're unfortunate enough to be near a hospital when your last days on earth approach, your doctor will make sure your $500-a-day deathbed has all the latest eletronic gear with a staff of strangers to hear your last words. But since those strangers are paid to keep your family away from you, you won't have anything to say. Your last sounds will be the electronic whistle on the cardiogram. Your relatives *will* participate: they'll pay the bill.

No wonder children are afraid of doctors. They *know*! Their instincts for real danger are uncorrupted. Fear seldom actually disappears. Adults are afraid, too. But they can't admit it, even to themselves. What happens is we become afraid of something else. We learn to fear not the doctor but what brings us to the doctor in the first place: our body and its natural processes.

When you fear something, you avoid it. You ignore it. You shy away from it. You pretend it doesn't exist. You let someone else worry about it. This is how the doctor takes over. We let him. We say: I don't want to have anything to do with *this, my body and its problems,* doc. You take care of it, doc. Do what you have to do.

So the doctor does.

When doctors are criticized for not telling their patients about the side effects of the drugs they prescribe, they defend themselves on the grounds that the doctor-patient relationship would suffer from such honesty. That defense implies that the doctor-patient relationship is based on something other than knowledge. *It's based on faith.*

We don't say we *know* our doctors are good, we say we have *faith* in them. We *trust* them.

Don't think doctors aren't aware of the difference. And don't believe for a minute that they don't play it for all it's worth. Because what's at stake is the whole ball game, the whole ninety per cent or more of Modern Medicine that we don't need, that, as a matter of fact, is out to kill us.

Modern Medicine can't survive without our faith, because Modern Medicine is neither an art nor a science. It's a religion.

One definition of religion identifies it as any organized effort to deal with puzzling or mysterious things we see going on in and around us. The Church of Modern Medicine deals with the most puzzling phenomena: birth, death, and all the tricks our bodies play on us — and we on them — in between. In *The Golden Bough,* religion is defined as the attempt to gain the favor of "powers superior to man, which are believed to direct and control the course of nature and of human life."

If people don't spend billions of dollars on the Church of Modern Medicine in order to gain favor with the powers that direct and control human life, what do they spend it on?

Common to all religions is the claim that reality is not limited to or dependent upon what can be seen, heard, felt, tasted or smelled. You can easily test modern medical religion on this characteristic by simply asking your doctor *why?* enough times. Why are you prescribing this drug? Why is this operation going to do me any good? Why do I have to do that? Why do you have to do that to me?

Just ask *why?* enough times and sooner or later you'll reach the Chasm of Faith. Your doctor will retreat into the fact that you have no way of knowing or understanding all the wonders he has at his command. *Just trust me.*

You've just had your first lesson in medical heresy. Lesson Number

Two is that if a doctor ever wants to do something to you that you're afraid of and you ask *why?* enough times until he says Just Trust Me, what you're to do is turn around and put as much distance between you and him as you can, as fast as your condition will allow.

Unfortunately, very few people do that. They submit. They allow their fear of the witch doctor's mask, the unknown spirit behind it, and the mystery of what is happening and of what will happen, to change into respectful awe of the whole show.

But you don't have to let the witch doctor have his way. You can liberate yourself from Modern Medicine — and it doesn't mean you'll have to take chances with your health. In fact, you'll be taking less of a chance with your health, because there's no more dangerous activity than walking into a doctor's office, clinic, or hospital *unprepared.* And by *prepared* I don't mean having your insurance forms filled out. I mean you have to get in and out alive *and* accomplish your mission. For that, you need appropriate tools, skills, and cunning.

The first tool you must have is knowledge of the enemy. Once you understand Modern Medicine as a religion, you can fight it and defend yourself much more effectively than when you think you're fighting an art or a science. Of course, the Church of Modern Medicine never calls itself a church. You'll never see a medical building dedicated to the religion of medicine, always the medical *arts* or medical *science.*

Modern Medicine relies on faith to survive. All religions do. So heavily does the Church of Modern Medicine rely on faith that if everyone somehow simply forgot to believe in it for just one day, the whole system would collapse. For how else could any institution get people to do the things Modern Medicine gets people to do, without inducing a profound suspension of doubt? Would people allow themselves to be artificially put to sleep and then cut to pieces in a process they couldn't have the slightest notion about — if they didn't have faith? Would people swallow the thousands of tons of pills every year — again without the slightest knowledge of what these chemicals are going to do — if they didn't have faith?

If Modern Medicine had to validate its procedures objectively, this book wouldn't be necessary. That's why I'm going to demonstrate how Modern Medicine is not a church you want to have faith in.

Some doctors are worried about scaring their patients. While you're reading this book, you are, in a sense, my patient. I think you *should* be scared. You're supposed to be scared when your well-being and freedom are threatened. And you are, right now, being threatened.

If you're ready to learn some of the shocking things your doctor knows but won't tell you; if you're ready to find out if your doctor is dangerous; if you're ready to learn how to protect yourself from your doctor; you should keep reading, because that's what this book is about." *(Reproduced by permission of Dr Robert Mendelsohn.)*

If medicine is a scandal, why isn't something done about it? Something is being done about it, but medicine has been a part of human culture for thousands of years and beliefs in it, like the beliefs in religion, change not by decree but by evolution, and evolution is a slow process. Entrenched medicine will change only when pressure outside forces it to. Meanwhile the old concepts persist. These concepts are engrained not only in the minds of doctors, but the minds of nearly everybody, they are a part of our culture, and it must be accepted that we are all products of our upbringing and training.

Medical training is based on the belief that there are many entirely different diseases, unrelated to each other, which for some reason or another concentrate their attention on human beings, as likely to 'attack' any one person as another. Often the person affected is referred to as a 'victim' of the particular disease, which must be carefully diagnosed according to the symptoms so that specific medical measures can be applied to the symptoms to remove them. Thus, whether a disease is categorized as an infectious disease or a metabolic disease, allopathic (conventional) medicine is directed more at the removal of the symptoms than to the removal of the underlying cause of the condition leading to the symptoms.

Enormous amounts of medicinal drugs are prescribed and if one doesn't work then another is tried, more often than not accompanied by half a dozen others which for some reason or other the doctor hopes will do some good. Chronically-sick patients may traipse from doctor to doctor, all the while deteriorating under the influence of the drugs accumulating in and poisoning their system. And all the while, the drug companies make bigger and bigger profits, generously supporting medical research devoted to producing more and better drugs, and spending large sums to keep the medical fraternity suitably brainwashed and drug-orientated.

When, as we have seen, the real causes of the diseases of civilization can be so clearly identified, why is the medical profession still so confused and ignorant? When will doctors begin to treat causes and not effects? Never, if the drug industry has its way.

Doctors who step outside the narrow protocols of established medicine are labelled crackpots by their peers. Even Linus Pauling, the recipient of two Nobel Prizes, could not get a research grant because his work with Vitamin C was too unconventional (not to mention that Vitamin C is not a patentable drug), but at least he has influenced a lot of medical thinking. People who do this sort of research find it hard to get their research papers accepted for publishing by medical journals. Doctor Gerson and many others like him have had and are still having the same trouble. It is a 'Catch 22' situation in which the researcher, denied research funds, cannot produce enough scientific evidence to carry weight, and so his research reports are labelled 'anecdotal' and therefore valueless.

It is a common ploy of the 'establishment' to emasculate research that does not fit their design by calling it 'anecdotal', by which they imply that it is worthless and should be ignored. Thus, the ordinary medical fraternity and the people who depend on them are kept in a continuing state of ignorance, their hopes for a better world dependent on the cult of high technology and the 'magic bullet' drugs and vaccines continually promised but never delivered.

'Anecdotal evidence' and 'Unproven methods'

Because there is so much chance of error when evaluating new concepts in medical methods, theories are not accepted as facts until rigidly tested under scientific scrutiny. Tests may involve the participation of many patients under treatment who are compared with others and so on, and may take years to complete. These tests are compared with the results of other tests until finally a concept may gain wide acceptance. Such tests may cost many thousands or even millions of dollars to conduct.

Thus medicine has become 'scientific' instead of the art it was once considered to be, and if new concepts or new evidence of any nature are presented, unless they are supported by 'scientific' studies they receive scant attention. Such 'unscientific' evidence, no matter how compelling, is called 'anecdotal' and not worth the paper it is written on.

People often ask "If natural therapies are so good, why aren't they being used everywhere?" The answer to this question is: because there is no money to be made in natural health and therefore the people who would dearly love to present scientific evidence as to its merits can rarely get the financial support needed to carry out the required studies to prove their argument.

Although most doctors have the welfare of their patients at heart, the overriding force in a drug-orientated medical profession is money, and therefore over many years there have been forces within the medical profession directed against the practise of natural hygiene and diet as a means of eliminating disease. There is no money to be made by the drug companies out of healthy people and none to be made selling sick people green vegetables and fruit.

Thus, for this and other reasons more obscure, the purveyors of 'Natural Health' have been labelled as quacks and all their brilliant accomplishments been dismissed and ignored by the use of the old ploy of calling them 'anecdotal'.

The Gerson Institute, now run by Gerson's daughter, Charlotte, in Bonita, California, has achieved by the use of the Gerson diet much better results with patients suffering from all the degenerative diseases than has the Pritikin Center, but whereas the Pritikin system has become famous, still the Gerson Institute struggles for recognition. Dr Gerson's presentations of cured cancer patients to the Senate Select Committee in Washington in 1946 and his fifty cases detailed in his book *A Cancer Therapy* could scarcely be called anecdotal, but were still ignored by the medical establishment, just as was the favorable investigation of Dr H. Hoxsey's cancer clinic in Texas at about the same time.*

The Gerson Institute has many times invited and then challenged the various medical institutions in the USA to investigate their claims of 'curing the incurables' — cases of cancer, leukemia, multiple sclerosis and so on — but the medical professionals just don't want to know. At a convention in San Diego in October 1981, the Gerson Institute presented one hundred fully recovered 'incurable' patients, half of them patients previously labelled as having terminal cancer, together with their medical case histories, and issued a formal challenge for any authority, medical or otherwise, to investigate these cases. They didn't even get a reply.

The American Cancer Society, the AMA, and the rest of the 'Medical Establishment' consider any treatment of cancer other than the orthodox medical treatments of surgery, radiation and chemotherapy, to be quackery, regardless of the fact that dietary and orthomolecular methods succeed infinitely better than their methods. Not only do these bodies refuse to even investigate alternative methods, worse than that they have exerted their powerful influence in government circles to have alternative cancer therapies declared illegal. As a result doctors practising alternative methods and gaining better results than conventional therapies

**You Don't Have To Die* by Dr Harry S. Hoxsey.

are still persecuted and subjected to de-registration and even imprisonment. This is why patients, given up as hopeless, have to travel to Mexico for the only treatment that offers them hope. That the natural therapy cancer patients can get in Mexico is supervised by fully qualified medical doctors and that the therapy achieves far better results than the orthodox methods, is ignored by the medical establishment which denigrates the results as being anecdotal and unproven.

By calling natural therapies unproven, the establishment of course implies that their orthodox methods are in fact proven. It all depends on what you mean by proven. Surgery, radiation and chemotherapy have been proven to be traumatic, disfiguring failures and further proven to be so by the relentless increase in cancer deaths as each year goes by.

That such negative forces endangering humanity can be overcome was demonstrated by Nathan Pritikin. Pritikin realized that to have his work accepted by the medical establishment he would have to follow conventional pathways. All his recovered heart-cases would impress nobody unless he presented the cases scientifically in the approved fashion. This cost Pritikin a lot of money, but with the help of dedicated doctors and others, he got his evidence together, and against a lot of opposition from the establishment (particularly in view of the fact he was not even a doctor), he forced his concepts to be accepted. Nathan Pritikin's contribution to humanity was not the Pritikin diet because there were already better diets to choose from; his contribution was beating the 'forces of agnosticism' (as Dr Warburg called them) and in doing so Pritikin displayed the highest qualities of intelligence, courage and determination that could be possessed by any human.

Pritikin's success lay in getting his well-proven accomplishments out of the "anecdotal" class into the "scientific" class where suddenly it became respectable. Being anecdotal is like coming from the "wrong side of the tracks" — nobody wants to know you.

One of Nathan Pritikin's predecessors in the field of nutrition and health was Dr Denis Burkitt of England who spent twenty five years of his medical career researching in Africa. Dr Burkitt is the man who gave his name to the rare form of cancer known as 'Burkitt's lymphoma' and who made the world aware of dietary fiber. Burkitt knew what it was like to be labelled a crackpot and to have his reports labelled as 'anecdotal'. Years later, at the Pritikin Center's annual conference in Santa Barbara, California, he said: "anyone who rejects evidence simply on the grounds that it is anecdotal would stand on the end of a jetty with a lifebelt in his hand and watch a man drown, not throwing the lifebelt because there was no scientific evidence that it would save the man's life."

Spontaneous remissions — medical mysteries or natural healing?

Chronic, 'incurable' diseases such as cancer, multiple sclerosis and arthritis usually follow a course, getting worse with the passage of time. At times during the course of the disease the patient's symptoms may lessen or go away for a while and the disease is said to have 'gone into remission'. What does this really mean? Is the disease some sort of attacker which has taken a rest from its efforts to destroy the patient's body?

Of course not. Disease means that the body is not functioning properly, so when the disease 'goes into remission' it simply means that the body has recovered, or partly recovered its normal function. It means that some factor adversely affecting the body's metabolism has diminished or has been removed and that the body's natural recuperative powers have restored it towards its natural state which is health.

When doctors say that their mission in life is to fight disease it shows that they don't understand what disease is. To eliminate disease you don't have to fight anything, you merely restore a favorable condition of blood chemistry within the body whereupon the body — of its own accord — restores itself to health.

If this simple fact is understood it can be realized that the term 'remission' is incorrect because it is not descriptive of what is happening. Remission implies that an entity which is trying to harm someone has relaxed its efforts. But no such entity exists. A better way to describe the situation would be that the patient's health is improved. Or, in the case of complete recovery, 'the patient is fully recovered'.

It could be argued that the act of destroying germs is fighting disease, but that argument is not quite true either, because the real disease is the lowered condition of the patient's health which allowed the germs to become active in the body. Killing germs is what the body should be doing for itself, and unless proper health is regained there soon will be another infection to take their place.

It could also be argued that cancer is something which exists and which must be fought. This is a better argument but even though in some cases the destruction of a tumor may improve the patient's chances, the fact still remains that the cancer only started in the first place because of defective chemistry within the body and because the immune system was too weak to prevent its spread, and so for the patient to recover good health the same basic rules of diet and lifestyle must be followed as with any other disease problem. No matter how much the cancer growth is attacked with surgery etc, the prime essential is to restore a favorable *milieu interieur* within the body so that the restorative powers of Nature can get to work.

When doctors observe the symptoms of disease go away consequential to medical treatment, the patient is described as cured. But medicine cannot 'cure' anything, it may well make the patient feel better, which mental state together with the doctor's reassurance and with rest may allow the body to restore itself — but cure — no, there is no such thing.

When the symptoms of, say, cancer or arthritis or multiple sclerosis disappear entirely of their own accord — an event most unusual — the event is called in medical parlance 'spontaneous remission' and is placed in the category of unexplainable phenomena. If instead of putting spontaneous recoveries aside as unexplainable, efforts were made with an open mind to explain them, the secret would reveal itself just as it did to Dr Gerson when his migraine patient's lupus healed. Inner chemistry! But medical training places the mind in a straight-jacket. A recent news report described how a 'terminally' ill AIDS patient after a short while on a raw vegetarian diet became fit and well. A doctor, when asked to comment, replied that the diet had nothing to do with it, the patient had had a spontaneous remission! Of course it was a spontaneous remission, but did the doctor think the fairies had contrived it?

In his book *Victory Over Cancer* author Cyril Scott quotes surgeon Hastings Gilford stating in 1925: "Though cancer is so commonly regarded as inevitably fatal, many cases are recorded of its spontaneous disappearance — and nothing can be more certain than that these recorded cases are very few in comparison with those which are unrecorded." Dr Gilford went on to list the names of many eminent men who have testified to spontaneous 'cures' of cancer. Among the names were Paget, Brodie, Muller, Sauerbruch, Gleitmann, Rohdenburg and Lomer. Lomer had recorded 213 cases and Rohdenburg 302.

Commenting on the fact of spontaneous remission of cancer, Dr Georgina Luden of the USA said: "The importance of this fact cannot be overestimated. It is a proof positive that the human body can wage a winning fight against malignancy under the most untoward conditions. Since outside aid had proved useless, the victory must have been won by inside means. Changes in the body chemistry resulting from increased or renewed activity of organs by which the chemical condition in the body is regulated, seem to be the only available explanation, since the chemical composition of the blood must influence the body cells."

Now that is a profound statement for a doctor to make. Of course the chemical composition of the blood influences the body cells — it is the be-all and the end-all of their entire existence.

Sir Alexander Haddow, a past leader in cancer research, said the key lay in finding out why spontaneous remissions occurred. Of course he was right. With any disease 'spontaneous' or 'natural' remission is the only true 'cure'; and of course prevention, in the first place, is better than cure. That is the entire purpose of changing the diets of sick people, regardless of what their disease may be called. The body cares not what the name of its disease may be, all it wants is a pure, clean blood supply, whereupon it 'spontaneously' restores itself to health — just as explained by Professor Bernard one hundred years ago.

The future of medicine

There are signs that a gradual awareness of the importance of nutrition is dawning within the medical profession, an awareness forced upon it by persevering people like Nathan Pritikin. In 1982 a comprehensive report called 'Diet, Nutrition and Cancer' was issued by the US National Research Council. The report was prepared by a committee of people from the National Academy of Science, the National Academy of Engineering and the Institute of Medicine. Although the report revealed a lamentable lack of comprehension of the subject, it did in fact demonstrate that nutrition was a significant factor in the origins of cancer. Note that the report emanated from outside the medical profession, as has a recently released book in Australia called *Diet, Health and Disease in Australia,* written by a number of doctors and produced by the Australian Academy of Science.

The research for both of these books obviously did not extend far outside conventional circles. In relation to cancer the lack of knowledge was lamentable, as was the lack of knowledge of diabetes and other disease problems as described in the Australian book.

Inadequate as these books may be, it is gratifying that they have appeared at all; it shows that some doctors are at last breaking free of their mental shackles.

In his book *Man The Unknown* the great physician and philosopher Alexis Carrel said: "Unless the doctors of today become the dieticians of tomorrow then the dieticians of today will become the doctors of tomorrow." Maybe this is starting to happen. Evolution is a slow process, and bearing in mind that it took hundreds of years for people to accept that the world was round, I suppose we should not complain too much.

In defense of doctors

In criticizing others one must always put oneself in their position and remember "There, but for the grace of God, go I." And so in defense of doctors with all their ignorance of the 'outside world', this chapter concludes with an explanation by Dr G. T. Wrench of England contained in the introduction to his book *The Wheel of Health,* published in 1938.

> "It should be clearly understood that a doctor is one so saturated with people's illnesses and ailments that, if thoughtful, he is almost forced to look upon life as something heavily burdened by these defects.
>
> I shall myself carry with me the profound impression of the first months I spent in the hospital wards and out-patient departments many years ago. I had come from the vigorous and exuberant life of an English public school, where everything that really absorbed one's boyish interests was based on a glowing vitality and responsive health. After the penance of school hours there was plenty of time to let the muscles go — games, sports, ragging, bathing, or running and walking over untilled fields. All these things were of sunlight and wind or the raw cold, which made the blood snap round its course.
>
> Something of this life accompanies the early years of the medical student, but there is always about one the lure of the hospital work

to draw one to its consuming interests. One is caught in the meshes of the problems of disease, from which one will not be able to free the mind for the rest of one's life.

For impressions of youth are those that remain. They colour all one's thoughts and experience, they largely select that thought and experience. And the impression of the quantity of diseases and the suffering due to them is a tremendous one. I used sometimes to walk about London with my eyes down and with the question "Why?" upon my lips until I saw pictures of the many maleficent objects of pathology upon the pavements, so vivid was the impression which the microscope and the post-mortem room made upon me.

The effect was not one of depression; that is not the effect upon healthy youth. It was one which stimulated one like a stouter opponent than oneself at boxing. Here was truly a prodigious opponent, the problem of disease, why man is so affected.

After debating the question — Why disease? Why not health? — again and again with my fellow students, I slowly, before I qualified, came to a further question — Why was it that as students we were always presented with sick or convalescent people for our teaching and never with the ultra-healthy? Why were we only taught disease? Why was it presumed that we knew all about health in its fullness? The teaching was wholly one-sided. Moreover, the basis of our teaching upon disease was pathology, namely, the appearance of that which is dead from disease.

We started from our knowledge of the dead, from which we interpreted the manifestations, slight or severe, of threatened death, which is disease. Through these various manifestations, which fattened our text-books, we approached health. By the time, however, we reached real health, like that of the keen times of public school, the studies were dropped. Their human representatives, the patients, were now well, and neither we nor our educators were any longer concerned with them. We made no studies of the healthy — only the sick.

Disease was the reason for our specialised existences. There was also a great abundance of it. Between its abundance and its need to ourselves its inevitability was taken for granted. Gradually, however, a question forced itself upon me more and more insistently. Had not some of this 'inevitability' attached to disease come about by our profession only viewing disease from within? What would happen if we reversed the process and started by learning all we could about the healthiest people and animals whom we could discover? This question pursued me with considerable constancy, but unfortunately I was not provided with that will which is a part of what I reverence so much — the genius of discovery. Those who possess it grip an idea and never let it go. They are as passionate for it to get on in the world as the mother is for her offspring; daring, as even weak animals do, to challenge hopeless odds on its behalf. After achieving a small local repute in research, all I did was to apply for scholarships, and in my applications I placed a subject of my own choice, to study the health of the healthiest people I could discover.

I did not, of course, succeed. My proposal was probably looked upon as ridiculous. To research in health was a complete reversal of the accustomed outlook, which was confined by the nature of the profession to different aspects of disease. For to the profession disease is the base and substance of its structure and health just the top of the pyramid, where it itself comes to an end. To propose reversing this was like asking one to stand on one's head to get the right point of view.

At any rate my applications came to nothing, though I was offered work upon the accepted lines. In this I had not the necessary faith, so I gave up research and went into practice. I remained interested in very healthy people and read what I could about them, but the work imposed by the war and by practice in the following years withheld me from anything more than an academic interest in the old question — Health; why not?

It was not until two years ago, when I had more leisure, that a vivid sentence in the writings of Sir Robert McCarrison thawed my frozen hope. The sentence was: "These people are unsurpassed by any Indian race in perfection of physique; they are long lived, vigorous in youth and age, capable of great endurance and enjoy a remarkable freedom from disease in general." Further study of his writings was very encouraging. Here was a research worker who researched in health and healthy people; in fact he presented to himself health as a problem, and produced answers to it, in some such words as the following: "Here is a people of unsurpassed health and physique, and here are researches into the reasons thereof."

In this way it will be seen we come as researchers straight to health without intervention, and to health in the full dictionary sense of the word of wholeness, namely, sound physique of every organ of the body without exceptions and freedom from disease. This is the knowledge which we all want to know. We want to know what is full health, whether the tremendous part illness and ailments play in modern civilized countries is really necessary and, if not, upon what primarily does health depend. We can ourselves attain to health — or at least with our modern skill in investigation we should be able to do so — if this full health exists in any part of our Empire today. We shall at least learn more about how to be healthy ourselves and how to bring healthy children into the world by studying successful human examples than we can by any other way.

By studying the wings of birds in flight we have made our machines carry us through the air. By studying one of the healthiest peoples of the world we might so improve our methods of health as to become a really healthy people ourselves. A research in health is really promising. Well, here is one. Let us see if the promise is fulfilled."

In Conclusion

It should be noted that this chapter, which so heavily denigrates the modern practise of medicine, is composed entirely from the observations and opinions of doctors and scientists. It concludes the same way, with the statements of three of the most distinguished physicians of the 20th century.

Dr William Roe (retired) of Nelson, New Zealand, the author of *Science in Medical Practise* (1984) in which he strongly criticizes modern medicine, said this:

"No more than a superficial acquaintance with anthropology, ethnology, or history is required for it to become apparent that the need to indulge in fantasy is deeply ingrained in man. Indeed it seems the most distinctive (and perhaps the most dangerous) characteristic of that species of the genus *Homo* we conceitedly label *Sapiens* is not his wisdom but his reluctance to admit ignorance. Rather than do so, he is prone to posit an hypothesis and, all too frequently in the absence of supporting evidence, comes to believe it. Thus are myths created."

In the same article, in discussing how the "scientific" method of acquiring information has displaced all others, Dr Roe said: "By starting from a false premise, a superstructure has been created which is, to a not inconsiderable degree, an iatrogenic* fantasy. The primary function of medicine has been transformed from a service to patients to a vocation and avocation for medical and paramedical personnel; iatrogenic disease has become a major problem and medicine has become big business. An urgent need exists to correct this imbalance, to restore the art of medicine to its former status."

Dr Kasper Blond, of England (referring specifically to cancer): "The problem of cancer must be considered as an insoluble medical problem because it is essentially a nutritional and social problem;** in other words, a problem of prevention.

"Such a problem cannot be solved by animal experiments, vaccines and drugs. Statisticians, pathologists, biochemists and doctors cannot solve social problems."

And finally to repeat the great Dr Alexis Carrel: "Unless the doctors of today become the dieticians of tomorrow, then the dieticians of today will become the doctors of tomorrow."

Dr Carrel said that in 1935, what about it, chaps?

*Iatric — relating to medicine or physicians.

**(As are all the rest — *Author.*)

CHAPTER TEN

Grains Are For The Birds

The population numbers of all creatures on Earth are limited by the resources of food and water available to them, and therefore remain fairly stable. Population explosions occur in various species when from time to time their natural food resources increase, but the numbers soon dwindle again when food becomes more scarce.

The population explosion of the human race commenced when primitive man learned to expand his resources of food by the use of technology.

Meat is not a natural food for primates but when early man learned the use of fire he soon found that animal flesh, revolting to him in a raw bloody state, could be rendered palatable by cooking it. This development provided a better chance of survival as man migrated out of the tropics, but introduced at the same time the curse of disease.

Grass seeds are not a natural food for primates either, because even though they contain nourishment, they also contain substances which are harmful. These harmful substances include enzyme inhibitors which are chemicals put there by Nature to prevent germination until favorable conditions exist. As explained earlier, these enzyme inhibitors prevent the digestive enzymes of animals from functioning, thus rendering matured, dry seeds (including nuts) indigestible unless they are first germinated. The only animals to which this restriction does not apply are the seed eating birds equipped with a crop in which the seeds, swallowed whole, remain until germinated after which time the bird can digest its food. But early man in his constant search for food learned that he could use seeds for food when they were ground up and cooked. The grinding exposed the starch so that man's starch-splitting enzymes could work on it, and the cooking destroyed the enzyme inhibitors that otherwise would have stopped the enzymes' action. This development again greatly enhanced man's chances of survival, because not only did it provide a new source of food, it was food which, in grain form, will keep to sustain people when other food is scarce. But as with the adoption of meat, there are drawbacks to the use of grains when incorporated in the human diet.

The human population explosion increased mainly in countries outside the tropics with the invention of farming which enabled primitive man to produce animals for meat and dairy products (dairy products being another unnatural food for man), vegetables, and most important of all, grain crops. By comparison, the production of fruit, man's natural food, became quite secondary, but this did not hinder the population explosion, even though the human life potential would always remain to a greater or lesser extent diminished by the use of unnatural food.

Man has been described as 'the thinking animal', 'the tool-making animal', 'the cooking animal', 'the destroying animal', and so on. He is all of these, but as his technology renders his food to be less and less natural, probably the best description of him would be 'the sick animal'.

Back to cereals. Cereals are grains of various kinds derived originally from the seeds of wild grasses. Wheat, corn, maize, rice, oats, rye and barley are all cereals. Cereals, having made the human population explosion possible, still form the basis of the diets of the majority of people on Earth. Cereals contain mainly starch which is a complex carbohydrate and therefore many people's main source of energy. Cereals contain considerable amounts of protein as well, far more than the human body requires.

As well, they contain small amounts of fat, and so it would appear that cereals provide complete nourishment, and to consider the fact that rice, wheat and corn sustain the vast populations of all the continents on Earth would seem proof enough.

But not all of these people fare well. Because of the deficiencies of vitamins and minerals in cereals, and the fact that they produce acid in the body, good health can only be maintained on them when the diet is supplemented with vegetables or fruit. The less the cereals are supplemented, the poorer the health and the shorter the life-expectancy of the cereal eater.

Apart from deficiencies which can be made up by 'balancing the diet', cereals have other drawbacks which cannot be counteracted and which cause harm in the body.

The basis of the Pritikin diet is complex carbohydrate, and for athletes and health conscious people today complex carbohydrate is the 'in thing'. The prefix 'complex' applied to carbohydrate means that the carbohydrate molecules are of a complex structure and this is the sort of carbohydrate — starch — which is contained in cereals. Sugars of different sorts such as fructose (natural fruit sugar), lactose (natural milk sugar) and glucose (the sugar used to feed the cells of the body) are simple carbohydrates. Manufactured refined sugar is sucrose, also of simple molecule construction.

Starch molecules are harder to digest because the complex molecules have to be broken down by digestive enzymes into simple molecules before digestion can be completed, whereas sugars are easily digested because the carbohydrate molecules are already in simple form.

Why then did Nathan Pritikin bestow his blessing on complex carbohydrates, food which taxes the body's digestive system? Pritikin's mission, first and foremost, was the reversal of coronary heart disease. This was uppermost in his mind and so his reasoning followed:

- We must lower fat, cholesterol and protein, the causes of

atherosclerosis and heart disease. To do this we must cut out foods of animal origin. We must become vegetarian.

- As most of the food we eat goes into the production of energy, if we cut out animal foods which provide most of the energy in the Western diet, as well as the protein, where then will we get our energy and sufficient protein?
- The only other suitable foods available are cereals, root vegetables, and fruits, because green vegetables are so low in food value that you would have to eat them constantly all day long like cattle do to get enough. We must therefore choose between starch foods (cereals and potatoes) and fruit, and consider green vegetables mainly as a source of vitamins and minerals.

So far Pritikin's reasoning was correct, but at this point his pre-occupation of eliminating atherosclerosis became an impediment. He knew that cholesterol and triglycerides (blood fats) were the two factors most implicated in atherosclerosis and he was determined that his diet should diminish these in the blood to as low levels as possible. Cutting out animal derived foods completely eliminated cholesterol and the harmful animal fats from the diet, but what about triglycerides from vegetable sources? Pritikin knew that concentrated sugar of any kind — refined sugar or even extracted natural raw sugar — entered the bloodstream too quickly, upsetting the normal blood sugar levels and resulting in the production of triglycerides, his number two enemy. His reasoning logically continued:

- If out of our two remaining sources of energy and protein, one of them contains sugar, a substance which elevates triglycerides, we cannot entertain it as a principal source of nourishment.
- We must therefore severely ration fruit because of its sugar content and rely almost entirely on cereals to provide our energy and protein.

What was the outcome of this reasoning? It was a great outcome; Pritikin first of all eliminated his own atherosclerosis and then proceeded to eliminate the atherosclerosis in the bodies of thousands of people who followed his teachings.

This is how the current rage on complex carbohydrate started and why companies who make wholegrain bread, pasta, cookies and crackers are doing so well.

But the reversal of heart disease and its associated problems is not the be-all and end-all of health and longevity. There are other things to consider besides restoring good circulation. Unsticking the blood is only the first step in optimizing health, the second step is to get the blood's chemistry right. Pritikin had taken the lipo from lipotoxemia but much toxemia still remained. **When he grouped the natural sugars contained in fruit in with other sugars, Pritkin had made a fatal mistake.**

The sugar in ripe raw fruit is man's natural food, it is digested without strain and the wastage of enzymes, and when fruit is consumed raw and whole there is no effect on triglycerides other than to stabilize them at their natural levels. Fruit is the perfect source of energy and contains just the right amount of protein and fat to suit the human system. Fruit is appealing to the sight and appealing to the taste; Nature did not give humans a 'sweet tooth' for nothing.

On the other hand it could never be said that grains were a natural food for man. Imagine you are holding some dried wheat in your hand. Does the thought make your mouth water? You would have to be starving to death before you'd eat it! And if you did eat it, what do you think would happen? You would get indigestion, and most of the wheat would pass through you undigested. It would remain undigested for two reasons: firstly, your digestive enzymes could not penetrate the cellulose surrounding the starch cells to begin with, and secondly, should the starch somehow be exposed to them the enzymes still could not do much work because of the enzyme inhibitors that exist in all seeds and nuts once the seed is no longer green.

Okay, so man learned long ago he could digest grains if he first heated them. Heat bursts the cellulose skin covering the starch and at the same time destroys the enzyme inhibitors. Now imagine a hungry man sitting at table waiting for his dinner. His wife hands him a plate of hot wheat grains saying: "Here you are dear, I have removed all the nasty enzyme inhibitors and the starch is exposed to perfection." Nobody would be that silly. So, determined to feed her husband grain because she has read he should eat some complex carbohydrate, she discovers pasta. She cooks him spaghetti and hands him a plate of it. He throws it at her. She bursts into tears and goes home to mother. Her mother explains that not only must pasta and other grain products be cooked but they must somehow or other be flavored as well because they have no flavor of their own, and on their own have no appeal to the senses either of sight, smell or taste.

To eat oatmeal for breakfast you need to sweeten it with sugar, honey or fruit. Some people salt it in the cooking as well. Bread or toast you need butter and jam or pickles or something else to flavor it. They give unruly prisoners bread and water for punishment. Freshly baked bread can be delicious but you wouldn't eat it on its own. Crackers need salt. Spaghetti needs meat sauce or tomato sauce, garlic etc. Cookies and cakes have to be sweetened.

Most starch foods are difficult to digest, the degree of difficulty varying with the amount of ptyalin (amylase) in the eater's saliva and how thoroughly the food has been chewed. Nature arranged for amylase, the starch splitting enzyme, to be present in human saliva (where it is called ptyalin) to commence the breakdown of starch straight away on eating because starch is so hard to digest. The starch which Nature was providing for was the starch contained in fruit and vegetables. When fruit which is not quite ripe is eaten it does not taste sweet enough because the carbohydrate in it has not yet changed into sugar. Nature would prefer you to eat ripe fruit, but should you eat it unripe you will find you must chew and chew before you can swallow it. This chewing ensures plenty of ptyalin gets to work on the starch and as the starch starts to break down into sugar (maltose) under its influence, gradually the pulp tastes sweeter, and that's when you swallow it. You don't need to do all this chewing with sweet ripe fruit, it goes pretty well straight down and digests with ease, whereas if you didn't thoroughly chew the unripe fruit you would get indigestion.

The high "glycemic rating" of bread has already been explained. Bread digests very rapidly because, eaten dry, it demands thorough chewing which mixes it well with saliva so that the ptyalin gets straight to work on the starch. Lightly toasted bread digests even faster. Bread therefore may digest too rapidly and upset blood sugar levels, but in a different form, such as fried in fat, it will be hard to digest. One way or the other, wholegrain or white, bread is at best a mediocre food capable of great mischief in the body.

When cooked starchy foods are made into a mush like oatmeal, cornflakes, spaghetti, pasta etc. and then flavored, the taste buds and salivary glands are fooled. A few chomps, it tastes good, and down it goes — oatmeal mixed with water and milk, cornflakes all wet with milk, pasta mixed with gravy and fat — where's all the ptyalin? There isn't any, so the starchy mess sits in the stomach for several hours still not digesting, because in the stomach there are no starch splitting enzymes secreted. Finally, the mess enters the main digestive tract which is simply not designed to handle unsplit starch and certainly not starch mixed with grease. So now the pancreas has to get into high gear, it has to somehow start breaking all this starch down, and this it does by pumping out more amylase to get the show on the road.

Evidence of the difficulties of digesting complex carbohydrates is the production of large amounts of gas which is expelled from the rear end and which at the Pritikin Center is the cause of great embarrassment to some and the subject of great humor to others.

Thus the complex carbohydrate is finally digested, so what's the problem? The problem is that the digestive system has to work too hard when any cooked food is eaten, and more so when the food is complex carbohydrate. Because the extra load is placed mainly on the pancreas, the organ which produces the primary digestive juices, the pancreas enlarges to cope with the unnatural demand. Compared with animals in the wild, the human pancreas as a percentage of total body weight, is from two to three times larger. This is because humans eat food mainly cooked, and it is the populations who subsist primarily on cereals that display the effect most. As already mentioned, Malays and Filipinos whose diets were composed mainly of rice were found to have pancreas weights on the average 50% greater than those of Americans. Tests with animals have shown that when rats are fed on laboratory food, supposedly composed of a perfect balance of nutrients, in a period of 155 days their pancreas enlarged by 30%. Other tests have shown that the pancreas is not the only organ affected, there being an enlargement of the liver and a decrease in weight of the pituitary and suparenal glands.

The Bantu natives of Africa whose diet is based on mashed corn and vegetables cooked in iron pots, while displaying little or no evidence of heart disease, have an extremely high incidence of liver disease, usually in the form of liver cancer which is the major cause of death among them. It has been conjectured that the liver disease among the Bantu is caused by the large amounts of iron from the iron cooking pots entering their bodies, but in view of the evidence, it would appear just as likely that the problem lies more in their poorly balanced diet and the subsequent wear and tear on the digestive enzymes and vital organs.

As mentioned, grains and grain products, regardless of whatever merits they may have, cannot provide complete nourishment because of their deficiencies, the main ones being of vitamins C, B and A, the amino acids lysin and cystin, and the minerals sodium, calcium and sulphur. All vitamins are essential to maintain normal metabolism and the integrity of the cells and tissues. On a diet of grains and cooked vegetables most of the vitamins are provided, but vitamin C, the most important vitamin of all for the maintenance of tissue integrity and immune system function, and the most easily destroyed by heat, will be deplorably lacking unless the diet is supplemented by a copious intake of fresh fruit. For the prevention of cancer and other tissue degeneration vitamin C intake should be generous. Dr Kasper Blond, the English cancer specialist, noted that the blood of cancer patients always displayed low levels of vitamin C.

Grains contain no vitamin C at all, and this fact alone is enough to disqualify them as food suitable for humans. Sprouted grains are a different matter, because as the germination of a seed progresses the seed changes from cereal form to vegetable form, the once dormant enzymes become very active, and vitamins, including vitamin C, are manufactured to sustain the growing plant. Dr Howell describes in his book *Enzyme Nutrition* (1985) how before the days of modern wheat harvesting methods, the wheat crop was cut and stacked in sheaves which would stand in the fields for perhaps some weeks before it was collected and threshed to take out the grain. During the time it was exposed to the weather, and by the time the grain was separated it would often have commenced to germinate a little and therefore offered better nutrition than the wheat as harvested today.

Wholegrains, beans and peas contain the harmful substance, phytic acid, in large amounts. This acid has the property of combining with minerals, especially calcium, iron and zinc to form insoluble compounds unusable by the body and thus diminishing further the nutritional qualities of these foods.

Studies made by various medical researchers, some as long as one hundred years ago, incriminate cereals, wheat in particular, in causing deposits of calcium salts in the tissues, especially in the arteries, which solidified and hardened them. This will be described later. Similar tissue degeneration was observed in Indian people whose diet consisted mainly of rice.

How cereals became 'health foods'

When many years ago the USA, Canada and Australia became the producers of vast amounts of wheat, it was cheaper for the European countries to import wheat than to grow their own, and this resulted in farming being devoted mainly to the production of animals and dairy products. During World Wars I and II, the imports of wheat were drastically reduced or cut off altogether, and in order to produce enough food it became necessary to cut down on livestock and devote farming to the production of wheat and vegetables. As the war years passed it was noted that death rates from heart attacks, cancer and other degenerative diseases fell dramatically subsequent to the severe rationing of meat, dairy products and sugar, only to rise again when these items became plentiful again after the war. The wartime diet was of necessity based on wheat products, potatoes and other vegetables, and the reputation of these foods as health foods was enhanced by the fact that on the wartime diet, health standards were noticeably improved. Austria is the only country in the world that requires autopsies of all deaths regardless of circumstances, and the statistics show there that in the years between 1939 and 1945 deaths from heart attacks decreased by 75%.

Thus it would appear that the low fat, low cholesterol, wartime diet in Austria had actually decreased the amount of heart disease there. But, according to Dr Broda Barnes MD, PhD, in his book *Solved, the Riddle of Heart Attacks* (1976) this was not the case. He says: "I have personally reviewed 70,000 autopsy protocols at Graz, Austria, carried out between the years 1930 and 1970. At Graz, heart attacks dropped 75% between 1939 and 1945, and it is true that people were not eating cholesterol foods during the war. However, the low cholesterol diet did not protect their arteries from hardening. A look at the arteries of the entire series of 2000 autopsies in 1945 revealed that the number of individuals with damage to their coronary arteries was approximately doubled in 1945, and the degree of damage to each one was about twice as great. In other words, the low cholesterol diet had not only failed to protect the arteries, but the damage was increased fourfold."

What can be deduced from this information? We know that, properly implemented, the Pritikin diet will permit the body to reverse artery disease. Animal tests have proven this, and the autopsy of Nathan Pritikin himself showed the arteries throughout his body to be clean and healthy. So two questions arise: Why were the arteries of the Austrians so diseased on their low fat and cholesterol wartime diet? And, given that they were, why did the heart attack rate drop by 75%? We are forced to the conclusion that the intake of cereal foods and potatoes, possibly salted, must not have been properly supplemented with fresh, raw, green salad, the way Pritikin supplemented his; and to answer the second question: simply that it is well known that on a low-fat diet the viscosity of the blood is low enough to permit reasonable circulation even when the arteries are almost totally blocked. It is significant that another review of Austrian autopsies showed that in 1958 the death rate from heart attacks was 700% higher than in 1944 when wartime stress was at its worst.

Allergies

When I told Nathan Pritikin of the problems I had experienced while on the Pritikin diet, and of my conclusions about grain products causing me harm he said that it must be that I was allergic to them, but I knew that I was not because I had eaten these things all my life without noticing any ill effects. It was only when I began to eat a lot of them that the trouble arose.

When a person experiences a noticeable upset subsequent to eating a particular food, they are said to be allergic to it. The upset is due to the fact that the substances of the food are not fully broken down by the enzymes in the digestive tract and are ingested into the bloodstream in a form to a greater or lesser extent poisonous to the body. Many people display allergic reactions to cereals, in particular wheat, because their systems cannot handle gluten which is the protein cereals contain. The foods responsible for most allergies are eggs, grain products and dairy products. 33% of all allergies are accountable to eggs and 30% to wheat.

The severity of an allergic reaction may vary for the same individual from time to time depending on the person's condition, the allergy sometimes presenting itself only when fatigue or stress is present. Such allergies have been alleviated by the intake of supplementary digestive enzymes, and this fact indicates that a lot more people would display allergies but for the power of their digestive enzymes. What I am saying is that eggs, wheat, dairy products and others are unsuitable foods for everybody, but do not always cause noticeable reactions because the body usually can break them down by drawing heavily upon its enzyme reserves.

That wheat in particular is harmful to the system is illustrated by the effect it has in the intestinal tract. Apart from the fact that wheat products are the main cause of coeliac disease, by which the intestines of an infant are irreparably damaged to make them allergic to cereals for life, similar but lesser damage may be caused to adults as well. Recent experiments by Dr E. W. Williams, University College of North Wales, showed that wheat protein is antigenic to rats. It causes hyperactivity in rats not used to them, and increased activity in those that are. In addition, Dr Williams found that the intestinal villi of the rats whose diet included wheat proteins, changed in shape from being long and slender to shorter and blunt. Similar villous atrophy had been observed in humans, he reported.

Thus it is a reasonable supposition that when eggs and dairy products cause allergic reactions in people it is because they are foods most unsuitable to the human system in the first place, and that these foods, full of cholesterol and fat, would be preferably left out of the diet whether the digestion can handle them or not. And in view of the demonstrated damage to the intestinal villi caused by wheat and other grain products, and in view of the so-called allergic reactions these products commonly cause, the same conclusion must be drawn about them too: grain products, whether they produce noticeable reactions or not, cannot be considered food suitable for the long term welfare of the human body.

Ossification of cells and tissues

Dr Charles De Lacy Evans, MRCS, PhD, of England in his book *How To Prolong Life — An Enquiry Into the Cause of 'Old Age' and 'Natural Death'* in describing old-age said: "The most marked feature of old-age is that a fibrous, gelatinous, and earthy deposit has taken place in the system; the latter being composed chiefly of phosphate and carbonate of lime, with small quantities of sulphate of lime, magnesia and other earths." His book went on to explain how these objectionable substances entered the body in varying amounts according to whichever foodstuffs comprised the diet, and how although the body excreted most of them there were always residues which gradually accumulated in the tissues. This subject will be enlarged upon in chapter 12 but in brief, Dr Evans' extensive research with both humans and animals revealed that in this regard cereals were the worst offenders, quote: "We now come to the cereals, in which we will include the leguminous seeds. The amount of earthy matter they contain depends upon the amount contained in the soil, or in the substances used as manure.

"The cereals constitute the basis of man's food; they mostly contain large quantities of mineral matter, and as a class are the worst adapted as a food for man, in regard to long life. Man's so-called 'staff of life' is, to a great extent, the cause of his premature death."

Cereals and Tooth Decay

Tooth decay (dental caries), common in civilized countries but practically unknown in primitive societies, is caused by the action of acid produced by bacteria in the saliva. These bacteria exist in everybody's mouth and are perfectly natural and normal. Whether they produce acid in the mouth or not depends on the sort of food eaten, and as mentioned previously in the description of cancer, the acid production is a consequence of fermentation. For fermentation to occur, the bacteria must be deprived of oxygen and this happens of course when food residues clog up the spaces between teeth. Sugar, alone, does not cause fermentation because it dissolves in saliva and does not deprive the bacteria of oxygen. Some foods readily ferment to produce a lot of acid and some foods do not. As well, the acid can to some extent be neutralized by saliva, but this depends on the quality of the saliva which in turn is dependent on the quality of the diet and the state of general body chemistry, so that some people are more prone to tooth decay than others.

The following description is taken from a report produced by Dr P. H. Belding, a dentist from Iowa, and his brother Dr L. J. Belding, a physician of the U.S. Naval Academy, Annapolis, following research on 1000 midshipmen at the academy in the 1930s:

"Staple products of the primitive diet, such as starch, rice, potatoes, molasses, orange juice, honey, sucrose and other sugars produce so little acid that it is difficult to see how they could be related to dental caries . . . On the other hand, particularly wheat and oats and to a lesser extent corn, were fermented with extreme rapidity with the production of large amounts of acid.

"Dental caries is a relatively specific disease occurring in those who partake of the modern diet; it is caused by the streptococci fermentation of specific cereal fractions."

Cereals and Head Colds

Another report from the 1930s, which appears to have escaped attention, followed a three year study on susceptibility to head colds by Dr Irwin Spiesman and Dr Lloyd Arnold of the University of Illinois:

"We found in our experience with dieting of these patients, that an over-indulgence of carbohydrates *(processed carbohydrates — Author)*, especially of the wheat-cereal variety, was most to be guarded against. Time and again we observed, after excellent results were obtained, that a return of the patient to an excess carbohydrate diet caused a recurrence of symptoms."

The study was of 63 people of all types. The report continued: "All of these people showed a greater tendency to get head colds the moment they included bread, cereals and other grain foods on their menu. Their resistance to colds was heightened enormously by eliminating grain foods."

Cereals and Arthritis

The association between grain products and arthritis has been mentioned already in chapters 1 and 6, but deserves yet another mention due to the frequency with which arthritis occurs to people on the Pritikin diet. Bread is the main offender, whether wholegrain or not, due to the fact it is not only acid forming but also results in elevated levels of blood fats (triglycerides), so making it a double barreled factor in arthritis. The reason bread affects the body differently to other complex carbohydrates is that, being dry, it mixes well with saliva and so digests too rapidly.

The Tarahumara Indians

Intent on demonstrating his diet to be the best in the world, Nathan Pritkin in his books uses the Tarahumara Indians of Northern Mexico as examples of perfect health and vigor attained on a diet almost the same as the Pritikin diet. The Tarahumaras, he said, subsist on a diet of mainly corn, pinto beans and other plant foods and fruit, with only a little animal protein and about 10% of the calories as fat, then went on to describe how this diet contained all the essential nutrients in more than adequate amounts.

The proof of such a diet, he claimed, was the fact that the Tarahumaras displayed virtually no incidence of heart disease, diabetes, high blood pressure or cancer, and have incredible physical endurance, being able to run a hundred miles a day five days in a row, carry heavy weights long distances, and so on. Pritikin said further: "Their diet, rich in grains, vegetables and fruits, is as close as science has come to optimum nutritional balance for human beings."

But the Tarahuramas on this "optimally balanced" diet fare no better than laboratory rats fed their "optimally balanced" prepared diet — in fact not as well. Laboratory rats appear to maintain good health when young, but if they are permitted to live out their lives they exhibit premature degeneration similar to senile humans, and die at a comparatively early age. Of all children born to the Tarahumaras, only one in five survives to five years, the others succumbing to malnutrition and disease, according to Dr William T. Jarvis, specialist in preventive medicine at the Loma Linda University in California. Moreover, those Tarahumaras who survive to adulthood and who are capable of great feats of endurance, don't live very long at all, the information — not documented — is that few live much past the age of 40.

There is little doubt that all the required nutrients do exist in the Tarahumaras' diet in "correct" proportions as tested in the laboratory, but the important thing is in what form do they exist, what else accompanies them, and how much wear and tear is caused during the body's attempts to utilise them?

Further evidence against cereals

Dr Rudolph Ballentine MD, USA — excerpts from his book *Diet and Nutrition* (1978).

"Some digestive diseases for example, known to be aggravated by wheat have been found to be based on an intolerance to gluten.

Certain persons with schizophrenia also seem to react adversely to wheat, and research has demonstrated that there is often overall improvement by putting such patients on a wheat-free diet. Again, it is suspected that gluten is the substance to which such people react, though other constituents of the wheat might also play a part.

"In India, where it has been a major part of the diet for many thousands of years, the ancient medical traditions ascribe special and unique properties to wheat. It is said to be particularly prone to produce growth, thus being suitable as a food for children. It is also prescribed for convalescents, but traditional physicians are wary of its growth producing tendency in adults and suspect it of aggravating the tendency to develop cysts and other benign growths and tumors in the body."

"Phytic acid is a phosphorous compound found in most plant foods but in especially large amounts in whole grains, beans and peas. It has the property of combining with minerals, especially calcium, iron and zinc to form insoluble compounds which are carried out in the stool. It was noted long ago that foods high in phytic acid can lead a dog to rickets, a disease that stunts the skeletal growth of children, causing deformities of the head, chest and limbs, or which can cause enough softening in the bones of adults that they break even during normal use. Bread with added bran, for example, has been associated with calcium deficiency and rickets in certain villages in Persia."

"The refining of flour can drastically change the content and proportion of other vitamins, minerals, protein and even in some cases, toxic contaminants. Zinc and cadmium, for example, are both found in wheat. While zinc is essential, the cadmium is toxic, and exerts its negative effects by replacing zinc in strategic enzymes which are thereby incapacitated. Thus the ratio between zinc and cadmium is very important, but zinc is concentrated more in the outer layers of the grain while cadmium tends to be found in its center. Milling, then, selectively removes the zinc, while leaving the cadmium."

Dr Herbert Shelton, San Antonio, Texas — excerpts from *The Hygienic System Vol II, Superior Nutrition,* fourth edition (1956)

"Cereals, after Ceres, goddess of the harvest, are grains. Oats, wheat, rye, rice, barley, millet and similar grass seeds, used as foods, are denominated cereals. They grow and mature in short seasons, can be grown in parts of the world that have short growing seasons, will grow almost everywhere, may be produced with a minimum of effort and will keep almost indefinitely. For these reasons they have been the mainstay of whole populations, despite the many objections that may be offered to their use.

"It is necessary to sound a warning against the use of grains in the Hygienic diet. At their best, grains are inferior articles of food and they certainly form no part of the normal diet of man. Every man, woman and child in the land will be better off by leaving them out of their diet."

"According to Berg the proteins of most seeds, and especially those of cereals, are especially characterized by inadequacy due to a lack of cystin and lysin. In like manner, it is a common characteristic of seeds, not only to contain an excess of acid, also to exhibit a deficiency of calcium. For lime is almost always present in the soil, so that seeds need not contain any more calcium than is requisite to provide for the growth of the first rootlet. In animal organisms, on the other hand, the need for calcium is very great. Cereals, consequently, quite apart from the fact that they contain an excess of acid, are about the most unsuitable food we can force upon the growing animal organism. The best proof of this is that even granivorous birds collect insects to nourish their young. The fledglings of the most strictly vegetarian birds are carnivora.

"Squirrels often are forced, from the scarcity of food, to eat cereals. They bite off the end containing the germ and eat this, leaving the rest of the grain."

"All experimenters seem to agree that the much vaunted cereal diet is inadequate. Funk, Summons, Pitz, Hess, Unger, Hart, Halpin, Steembock, Davis, Hogan, Mendel, Wakeman, Parsons and others of equal standing agree with Berg who agrees with Densmore. Oats are deficient in basic salts. Wheat is deficient in sodium and calcium, while the germ of the wheat is inadequate as a growth factor. Rice is deficient in salts, and especially in calcium, also in sodium and chlorine. They are all lacking in iodine."

"We have learned, says Berg, that all cereals have certain defects which may be looked upon as characteristic of these nutriments: As regards inorganic salts, they are deficient in sodium and calcium; they are also poorly supplied with organically combined sulphur and with bases generally; but they contain a superabundance of inorganic acid-formers and of potassium. The cereals are also poor in vitamins A, B and C, the poverty being more marked in proportion to the fineness of the flour. Finally, the proteins of the cereals are always inadequate; they are lacking to some extent in the ringed amino-acids, and are especially poor in lysin and cystin.

"It has long been known that when herbivora,* and still more when rodents, are fed exclusively on grain, acidosis rapidly ensues. In rabbits on a maize (corn) diet, for example, the acid urine contains far more phosphorus than is being introduced in the food, showing that phosphorus is being lost from the animal's tissues. Rats, again, can only endure an exclusive grain diet for a short period, speedily succumbing to such a regime."

"Cereals are about the most difficult to digest of any habitual

*Horses kept by man for various purposes and fed on oats and chaff live about 25 years whereas horses running on wild pastures live about 50 years.

sources of starch except beans and peas. They are difficult for the infant and growing child. They ferment easily and cause much gas and intoxication.

"Of all starch foods eaten by man, cereals along with legumes, are the least fitted to the capacities of his digestive organs and are also least well-fitted to meet the nutritive needs of his body. Babies fed on such foods have indigestion, colic, diarrhea, constipation, colds, hives, tonsillar and adenoid troubles, and even more serious difficulties. They develop poor teeth and are soon making their regular visits to the dentist for tooth repairs."

"Wheat is the most acid-forming of the cereals. Oats seem to have the worst effect on the teeth. Rice, which is probably the best of the cereals, is the staple article of food in the diet of more than half the world's human inhabitants. Cases of beri-beri in humans have been reported in which whole and not polished rice constituted the bulk of the diet."

"Green corn is not classified as a starch. Some of our State Agricultural Experimental Stations have shown that when green corn is picked it immediately begins to ripen and will accomplish as much of the ripening process in twenty-four hours as it would have done in several weeks on the stalk. So rapid is the transformation of sugar into starch that in twenty-four hours it is changed from an alkaline ash food to an acid-ash food.

Germinated grains make better food than dry grains. Grains 'in milk', that is, before they have matured, are alkaline foods, but the mature grains are acid."*

"Bread eating is one of the great curses of modern life. Made of cereals, largely de-natured, mixed with salt, soda, yeast, lard and other ingredients and subjected to a high degree of

*Fresh young corn tastes sweet because it contains natural sugar which later turns to starch. Eaten at this stage sweet corn is a good food.

temperature in cooking and then eaten three or four times a day mixed indiscriminately with all classes of food, bread is one of our chief sources of woe. Breakfast foods (de-natured cereals) are eaten in considerable quantities in almost every household. 'Health' food stores turn out more cereal products than all other products combined.

The advocates of whole cereals, in preference to the de-natured kinds, did their work too well. Vegetarians are usually great eaters of cereals. They would receive less harm from moderate amounts of meat."

"We may state a few conclusions about cereals from the above facts:

1. Cereals do not form any part of the natural diet of man and are not necessary for health and life. (I believe geologists and anthropologists are agreed that man did not become a cereal eater until late in his history.)
2. They are best omitted from the diet entirely and especially from the diet of infants and children.
3. Where they are eaten, only the whole undenatured unprocessed cereal should be taken.
4. They should form but a small amount of the diet and should be offset with an abundance of fresh fruits and green vegetables — properly combined.
5. To ensure the conversion of their starches into sugar they must be eaten dry and not as porridges and mushes."

Dr Oliver Alabaster, Associate Professor of Medicine and Director of Cancer Research, George Washington University Medical Center — excerpts from *What You Can Do To Prevent Cancer* (1985).

"*Some Epidemiological Evidence.* Only a few studies have examined the association of various types of carbohydrates with either cancer incidence (how many people get it) or cancer mortality (how many people die from it).

"A weak association has been found between dietary carbohydrate and cancers of the pancreas, the liver, the breast, the stomach and the esophagus. Let us look briefly at the evidence, some of which is difficult to interpret.

"Cancer of the Pancreas and Liver. In 1975 scientists reported a significant correlation between sugar intake and death from pancreatic cancer. At the same time, they failed to demonstrate any relationship between the incidence of the disease and sugar intake. Moreover, this limited observation was confined to women. (Armstrong and Doll 1975, *International Journal of Cancer* 15:617-31.) The same study also found a weak association between the incidence of liver cancer and the intake of potatoes (a rich source of starch). To my mind, these limited findings do not amount to a significant case against carbohydrates, although they deserve further study."

"Cancer of the Stomach. After studying mortality rates for stomach cancer in sixteen countries, it was found there was a rather striking direct correlation between the intake of cereal in the form of flour and the risk of death from stomach cancer (Hakama and Saxen 1967, *International Journal of Cancer* 2:265-68). However, only one other study of patients with stomach cancer has revealed an above average intake of starch (B. Modan, Lubin, Barrell, Greenberg, M. Modan and Graham, 1974, *Cancer* 34:2087-92)."

"Cancer of the Esophagus. Most attempts to demonstrate an association between dietary carbohydrate and cancer of the esophagus have failed. However, there has been one study which evaluated the dietary patterns of patients in Singapore who had esophageal cancer (de Jong, Breslow, Hong, Sridharan and Shanmugaratnam, 1974, *International Journal of Cancer* 13:291-303). Their diets were compared with those of a comparable group of patients who had other diseases. The results suggested that the patients with esophageal cancer had a higher consumption of carbohydrates such as bread and potatoes. Of course they may also have had a higher consumption of something else too, and were never asked. Alternatively, there is always the possibility that these patients were eating fewer protective fruits and vegetables *because* they ate more bread and potatoes. Conceivably, the problem could have nothing to do with starch at all."

"Zinc is an essential part of more than 100 enzymes, and is consequently essential for life. This metal is intimately involved in the growth and division of all cells, and therefore it has a great influence on your immune system — part of your defense against cancer. Any deficiency in your dietary zinc will reduce your production of cancer-fighting T cells (Frost, Chen, Rabbini *et al*, 1977, *Proceedings of Clinical Biological Research*, 14:143) which could increase your cancer risk.* On the other hand, there is

**Author's Footnote on Cancer:* The U.S. Government $200 million Multiple Risk Factor Intervention Trial (described in *The Health Revolution*), as well as confirming the expected relationship between blood cholesterol levels and heart disease at the same time showed a puzzling relationship between cholesterol levels and cancer (see J.A.M.A. February 20 1987). Among the 12,000 trial subjects the deathrates from cancer were about the same, regardless of their cholesterol levels, except for the group with the lowest levels (below 168 mg/dl or 4.3 m.mol.). This group, while suffering only a quarter the deathrate from heart attacks as the highest cholesterol group, had a deathrate from cancer almost 50% greater than all the others, causing some people to believe that low cholesterol levels could lead to cancer. But other tests had previously shown excess cholesterol to be carcinogenic. It didn't make sense.

We can make sense of it, however, if we put aside the low cholesterol levels themselves and devote our enquiry instead to the factors which produced the low levels. Pritikin showed that to achieve the cholesterol levels being discussed, all cholesterol-containing foods must be virtually eliminated from the diet and replaced with grains, vegetables and fruit. Most people, given this advice, greatly increase their intake of starch foods without much increasing the green vegetables and fruit, a fact which, in the light of the evidence, provides an explanation for the increased cancer. Cholesterol-lowering drugs could perhaps in some cases be involved too. Conclusion: Low cholesterol levels are desirable, starchy foods are undesirable.

evidence that excessive zinc may also be just as harmful.

Experimental studies have generally supported these findings, *with both high- and low-zinc diets appearing to increase cancer risk.*

The availability of zinc varies from one food to another, even if they contain similar amounts of zinc. Vegetarians can easily become zinc-deficient, and a diet that is high in dietary fiber can restrict absorption.

The best natural sources of zinc are seafood (especially oysters), eggs, liver and meat. Wholegrains such as wheat, rye, oatmeal and corn are poor sources because the zinc they contain is in a form that is relatively unusable."

Dr Emmet Densmore MD — excerpts from *How Nature Cures* (1891)

"We have come into possession of an old and rare pamphlet which is pregnant with striking scientific facts and philosophical deductions, and is remarkably pertinent to the main contention that bread, cereals and pulses are unwholesome foods for man. It consists of 'an enquiry into the cause of natural death, or death from old age; and develops an entirely new and certain method of preserving active and healthy life for an extraordinary period;' written by one S. Rowbotham, a surgeon who practised medicine in Stockport some fifty years since. Quote: 'The solid earthy matter which by gradual accumulation in the body brings on ossification, rigidity, decrepitude, and death, is principally phosphate of lime, or bone matter; carbonate of lime, or common chalk; and sulphate of lime, or plaster of Paris, with occasionally, magnesia and other earthy substances . . .

'We have seen that a process of consolidation begins at the earliest period of existence, and continues without interruption until the body is changed from a comparatively fluid, elastic, and energetic state, to a solid, earthy, rigid, inactive condition which terminates in death . . .

'The question now arises, what is the source of the calcareous earthy matter which thus accumulates in the system?'

'Common table salt, which is used in the preparation of almost every kind of food contains a fearful amount of calcareous, earthy matter, and is productive of very great mischief to the animal economy . . .'

'Bread (from wheaten flour), when considered in reference to the amount of nutritious matter it contains, may with justice be called the staff of life; but in regard to the amount of earthy matter, we may with equal justice pronounce it the staff of death.'

'Bread and potatoes constituting so large a proportion of the diet of the working classes, and containing so large a quantity of earthy matter, must inevitably render them more liable to disease and premature old age and death. And so it is found that the rate of mortality among the poor is much greater than among the rich, as the following table will show' . . ."

Monsieur Gubler, Professor of Therapeutics, Paris College of Surgeons (*Annales d'Hygiene,* Paris 1877, 2nd Ser. Vol. 48).

"The title of this communication sufficiently indicates that I do not here submit a definite solution to the problem, but simply some personal views, and a suggestion of a new method to be followed in the study of this difficult and interesting question of atheromatous degeneration.

"As age progresses, and under the influence of conditions still imperfectly determined, the inner wall of the arteries, supple and elastic in its normal state, thickens gradually and becomes indurated in such a manner as to offer, to the exploring finger, similar resistance to that of a bird's feather or the windpipe of a chicken, according as the degeneration is uniform in circular zones alternately with rings relatively healthy.

"By anatomic examination it is found that the thickening and induration of the vascular membrane is due to an accumulation of a whitey yellow and granulous and fatty substance, but essentially of mineral composition, the greater part of which is represented by the carbonates and earthy phosphates.

"This degeneration spares no one and affects all classes, but in a manner very unequally; indeed the contrast is something astonishing in this respect between the well-to-do and the working classes, between town and country people, the difference being entirely to the advantage of the first. While among those high in the social scale, supple arteries are to be noted until the approach of confirmed old age, in the inferior classes on the contrary, arterial induration often shows a striking precocity. Whence comes this strange disparity?

"It seemed to me that the nourishment, so different in the cases respectively of each class, poor and rich, country and town, would be able to furnish us with a satisfactory explanation of the facts noted. While the one class live principally on flesh (their favorite vegetables — mushrooms, truffles, asparagus — are themselves largely provided with the nitrogenous principle), the other class is sustained on vegetable substances, bread, potatoes, cabbages, salads and bean species, as well as fruits, forming the basis of their food.

"Now meat and other albuminous substances contain very little mineral elements; while the pulses and the fruits are well supplied with them. It is the leaves of plants that possess the function of condensing and retaining in their tissues the mineral matter in solution, in the ascending sap, and these organs, in decaying, yearly restore to the soil the earthy salts the plants have received. Such is the physiologic reason for the enormous proportion of earthy matter which the consumption of green portions of plants (and consequently of the pulses) introduces into the human economy, and into that of the herbivorous animals.

"The correctness of these views may be easily verified. If, as I think, the cretaceous incrustations of the arteries have their origin in the earthy matters supplied in a vegetarian regime, concurrently with drinking water charged with earthy salts, they will be more frequent, more premature, and more serious in chalky districts. Well, Dr Leblanc tells me he has been struck by the prevalence of this morbid state among the peasants of l'Orleans. On the other hand, in a region absolutely devoid of lime, and where the fowls can scarcely make shell for their eggs, hardening of the arteries is noted only in those of advanced years."

Some conclusions about grains

When first I started to read the 19th century accounts by Dr Rowbotham and Professor Gubler comparing the life expectancy of the poor and rich in England and France, I said to myself, "I know what is coming: the working class on their simple diet outlived the rich who indulged all the time on foods full of fat and cholesterol."

But I was wrong, and very surprised. Indeed the rich experienced the soft and mushy artery closure, known today as atherosclerosis as old age approached; but at a much earlier age the poor people who subsisted largely on bread and potatoes, experienced hardening of the arteries and their life expectancy was on the average much shorter.

At the turn of the century hardening of the arteries was the more common form of artery disease and was referred to as arteriosclerosis. Since then however, working class people have become more affluent and, having adopted the diet that once only the well-to-do could afford, now live longer and commonly suffer atherosclerosis, the soft and mushy blockage of the arteries. Despite this change, however, the death rate today from degenerative diseases is still higher among the 'blue collar' workers because the better educated classes have become more aware of the dangers in the diet of affluence.

Somewhat confused at first that artery disease could result in the absence of cholesterol and fat, it was enlightening to read Dr Broda Barnes' account of the same thing occurring in Austria on the wartime diet there based on grains and potatoes. As Dr Herbert Shelton said, "The advocates of whole cereals in preference to the de-natured kinds, did their work too well. Vegetarians are usually great eaters of cereals. They would receive less harm from moderate amounts of meat."

When arguments are presented against vegetarianism it is evident that many of the objections stem from the adverse effect of grains, pulses and legumes, all of which are seed-related foods which place great strain on the organs of digestion, and introduce undesirable substances into the body.

It should be clearly understood that grains are not vegetables, and a person who eats them is technically not a true vegetarian. In Nature, no animals eat grains apart from the seed-eating birds which are especially equipped with a crop to manage them and which are classified as granivorous, not vegetarian.

In brief, the objections to grains and grain products as foods suitable to the human system are:

1. They are deficient in a number of important nutrients.
2. They contain substances to some degree poisonous to the system.
3. They must be cooked in order to be digested which process further depletes their value and increases their pathological effect.
4. They place strain on the digestive system causing hypertrophy of the pancreas and unnecessary depletion of enzyme reserves while at the same time resulting in flatulence.
5. They are capable of damaging the intestinal villi causing the villi to atrophy.
6. They are acid-forming in the body, often to the extent of

causing arthritis and possibly cancer in the long term.

7. They are capable of causing allergy reactions such as dry skin, subcutaneous cysts, exacerbation of multiple sclerosis and schizophrenia.
8. They are antagonistic to the body's immune system and increase susceptibility to head colds and other infections.
9. They are the worst causative factor in tooth decay due to their tendency to readily ferment between the teeth, so producing the acid which destroys tooth enamel.
10. They are totally unsuitable for infants, causing in some cases permanent damage to their digestive organs.
11. Of all foodstuffs, they contain the highest levels of calcareous salts which gradually accumulate in the tissues and cells, including the arteries, to accelerate the process of aging.
12. Apart from antagonizing the digestive system and providing inadequate nutrition, they are absolutely tasteless and unappealing to the senses, being rendered edible only by cooking and artificial flavoring.

The Proof of the Pudding is in the Eating

If you are on the Pritikin diet or the Macrobiotic diet and wish to verify the disturbing information outlined in this chapter about cereals, there are two ways of doing it. First, you can spend a couple of years checking out all the sources of information, or second, you can abandon grain products completely for a week or so and see what happens.

Good quality fruit costs a lot more than bread or oats or spaghetti but you will find in the long run it is money well spent.

CHAPTER ELEVEN

Second Thoughts On Exercise

Everyone knows that exercise is good for you and that active people usually live longer and in better health than most. For instance, of the Hollywood stars of the 1940s and '50s, who have survived better than the 'hoofers' — the dancers — kept fit by constant physical exercise? Long after he-men like Errol Flynn, Gary Cooper, John Wayne and a host of others had gone to the big studio in the sky, Gene Kelly, Fred Astaire, Anne Miller, Cyd Charisse and Ginger Rogers were still going strong.

The man who taught the world to jog was Kenneth Cooper, whose book *Aerobics*, published in 1968, convinced millions of people that aerobic exercise was a sure-fire protection against heart attacks. It certainly convinced me; I read the book in Hong Kong on a stopover during my career as an airline pilot, and immediately having put the book down, set out to walk the streets for hours. Apart from improved fitness, my walking and running program broadened my education; instead of propping up various bars around the world, discoursing on trivia in my layover time, I had many new and interesting experiences, such as being attacked by dogs, apprehended by military armed guards, feeling the Golden Gate Bridge flex under my feet, and seeing the sun rise over the mountains of Tehran. Regarding physical fitness, I was once astounded to watch a Chinese coolie in Hong Kong, a small wiry man, pick up a huge basket of melons, put it on his head, and carry it up the steeply inclined gangplank from the deck of a junk to the wharf. I'd have thought it would take at least four men to lift such a load but he did it with relative ease, and without pausing for rest repeated the operation over and over for the half hour I spent watching him. Anybody picking on that little guy would be in for a big surprise, I thought to myself.

Anyway, I believed implicitly in Major Cooper's ideas about Aerobics and soon worked up to running six miles a day, rain or shine, Singapore, Sydney or San Francisco.

Checking my blood pressure records kept by the Department of Aviation over the previous 24 years, I was pleased to see the readings which had gradually risen in the 'normal' fashion to 145 over 85 (considered good for a man of 45), at my next medical had dropped to 128/80, and my resting pulse rate had dropped to 42. What's more, I never 'caught' colds when everyone else did and I knew I was in good shape, and better still, I felt I could eat and drink as I pleased without the slightest fear of heart disease, the disease that already had grounded several of my contemporaries. I preached Kenneth Cooper's gospel to all and sundry and actually got quite a few pilot converts, who like me, would welcome the healthy thirst long distance running gave one because of the added enjoyment it gave to the drinking of beer.

Thus I continued, fit as a fiddle, on a diet better than most but still with lots of fat and cholesterol. My weight was 145 pounds (66 kg), blood pressure perfect, no need for reading glasses, free of colds and free of the fatigue associated with long-haul flying. Nobody could say that Aerobic exercise was not beneficial — a man of 46 with a resting pulse rate of 42 had to be in a strong position — so in 1971 I wrote my first epistle for Qantas Airways, *Beat Heart Disease*, in which diet received only a brief mention.

When I met Nathan Pritikin in 1976 I believed that for the prevention of heart disease Aerobic exercise was 90% of the show and diet 10%, but Nathan soon convinced me it was the other way about — diet was 90% and exercise only 10%. This I still believe, although disagreeing with Nathan's views on diet.

With the heart attack deaths of so many endurance runners

since that time, the myth of endurance exercise as a guarantee against heart disease has become clearly exposed. A report issued in the *Journal of the AMA*, in 1982 entitled 'Incidence of Death During Jogging in Rhode Island from 1975 through 1980' indicated that death by heart attack was seven times more likely to be caused by jogging than during less vigorous activity. Some people now believe Aerobic exercise is actually harmful, and you would have to agree that a heart attack after a five mile run is every bit as harmful as one sitting in front of a television set.

To clarify this point it should be realized that heart disease and heart attack are not one and the same thing — one is the disease, the other is a symptom of the disease. Endurance exercise only appears to prevent heart disease because it tends to prevent the symptoms of it being displayed, but it must be admitted that if the onset of symptoms is delayed for a considerable time then this constitutes protection, even though only temporary. On the Western diet, arteries block up with fat and cholesterol whether you exercise or not. Aerobic exercise enables the arteries to expand to accommodate the demand for blood flow and it enables the body to more readily clear the bloodstream of fat deposited in it from the diet, which accounts for why athletes display lower blood viscosity and lower blood pressure than others. Obviously these effects provide much better circulation and therefore protection against heart attack.

But strenuous exercise has another effect and that is to temporarily increase the number of platelets in the bloodstream and to increase their tendency to clot. Platelets are cell-like particles which clump together to form blood clots to protect against bleeding in the event of injury, and clots so formed are readily dissolved again if not needed. The clotting and anti-clotting mechanism of athletes is highly efficient and it has been accepted that this is another advantage possessed by physically fit people. No matter how much this may be the case, when the athletes' arteries eventually block to a critical degree (which on the Western diet they inevitably must), then the increase in blood platelets resultant to exercise* can so increase the blood viscosity as to arrest circulation to critical areas of the heart. Relaxing blissfully after a good workout, the super-fit fifty year old, to everyone's amazement, has a heart attack. Had he not run that day he would have still been his usual 'fit' self,** but, on the other hand, had he not been so fit he may well have had his heart attack at forty-five.

Coffin corner

Jet planes fly high because in the thinner air there is less friction to overcome and so performance is better. However, there is a point where the benefits run out, and the airplane, although it is going very fast, finds itself in danger of stalling in the rarified air but cannot increase its speed to avoid the stall without running into the compressibility which accompanies high speeds. This point on the performance graph, jokingly referred to as "coffin corner", is a "catch 22 situation" similar to the one encountered by a fit athlete who chooses to remain on the Western diet. His improved performance lasts only until he sooner or later arrives at the "corner". However, should he survive the heart attack he can avoid the coffin part temporarily with a bypass operation, or, better still, to change his diet like Rolet de Castella† did and get out running marathons again.

How much exercise is sufficient?

Assuming you are not interested in long distance running or other

*Dr H. S. Sarajas of Helsinki noted that the platelets increased by up to double their base-line number after running as short a time as 30 minutes or after long vigorous walking. See 'Reaction Patterns of Blood Platelets in Exercise' reported in *Advances in Cardiology,* 18 (1976).

**In such a situation a heart attack could just as easily be precipitated by a high-fat meal or the onset of severe emotional stress. This is all explained in *The Health Revolution.*

†Father of world champion marathon runner Robert de Castella, Rolet suffered a stroke and heart attack at age 50. Two years later as a "cardiac cripple" he adopted the Pritikin diet and seventeen months later, completely free of medication, he completed the Victorian Marathon Championship in 3 hours 31 minutes. He has since run 30 marathons and has broken three hours for the distance. (See chapter 2, *The Health Revolution.*)

forms of endurance exercise (Aerobic exercise) and that you merely desire to maintain buoyant health and live long, what exercise is really necessary? We know that some sedentary people live to one hundred but that the majority of centenarians have been fairly active usually as manual workers until late in life., It is clear then that super-fitness is not required, regardless of a person's diet.

As explained earlier, the health and efficiency of the body is dependant on the health and efficiency of the body's individual cells and is determined therefore principally by diet. If the *milieu interieur* of the body is close to perfection it will follow that even with minimal exercise the body's various organs will function at an optimal level, the immune system will be powerful and the brain clear and active. The body may not be physically fit in the sense of performing arduous physical tasks, but will continue to perform otherwise at a high level free of fatigue and illness when many strong and super-fit athletes are laid up with influenza or something worse such as heart disease or cancer.

For the average person on the Western diet, which means nearly everybody — and more so for those who consume take-away meals — physical exercise must play a more important role in health maintenance because something needs to be done to clear the fats and toxins despoiling the bloodstream and extra-cellular fluid. Light exercise of any kind will help because it stimulates the flow of lymph (the extra-cellular fluid) which becomes sluggish when containing lots of fat in suspension. For a high level of health — meaning good circulation and a strong immune system — a person consuming the conventional high-fat diet needs the benefits of the 'Training Effect' conferred by Aerobic exercise, because without taking dietary accessories such as garlic or aloe-vera etc., only the training effect can clear the blood of fat and produce a reasonable *milieu interieur.*

The Training Effect

Aerobic exercise means exercise that places a fairly high demand upon the heart and lungs to provide the oxygen necessary to energize the muscles but at a level which can be maintained for periods of about ten minutes or longer. Such exercise brings about an improvement in body metabolism which Cooper termed the 'Training Effect'

In *The Health Revolution,* the physiological effects of exercise are discussed at length. Briefly, the Training Effect relates to the changes that take place in the cells of muscles used in the exercise program which enable them to more efficiently use fat as a source of energy and to more efficiently utilize the oxygen available to them. The most singular benefit bestowed by the Training Effect is to rid the blood of fat. From this single effect other great benefits flow; the red blood cells unstick, the platelets unstick, the red cells reduce in number because they are efficient again and the blood becomes oxygen enriched. The blood viscosity decreases and the heart need not exert itself so hard to pump the blood, and so the circulation is improved with less effort and the blood pressure falls because high pressure is no longer needed. At the same time, released from the embrace of fat, the white cells of the immune system become functional instead of semi-functional, and so an aerobically-fit person becomes infection-free. When sometimes athletes come down with infections, it is usually because they overstress themselves, a condition in which the immune system becomes depressed.

As a result of all these improvements the entire body works better, mental and visual acuity increase markedly, and it is easy to accept all these benefits as an indication of promised longevity, which to a great extent is a correct indication but not an infallible one.

Lymph circulation

Just as the blood circulation is impeded by the stickiness caused by excessive fat levels, so too is the flow of the lymph fluid which is fed by the bloodstream and upon which the body's cells depend for their livelihood. Whereas the blood circulation can be maintained by the heart pumping harder to increase the blood pressure, the lymph flow in the lymph vessels depends on physical stimulation to propel the fluid along. Like the veins of the blood circulatory system, the lymph vessels contain tiny valves which permit flow only one way so that the lymph finally returns to the bloodstream by a network of vessels similar to the veins. And for these vessels and the veins to conduct their function they must be squeezed from time to time by the movements of muscles and arteries adjacent to them. If the lymph is fat-free and free-flowing, its flow is easily accomplished but if it is sticky, then greater physical stimulation of the system is required. Any sort of exercise that involves general movement will achieve this, even getting up to answer the phone and so on. Light exercise such as calisthenics, while not capable of producing the Training Effect, will still be of great benefit simply by giving the lymph system a good clear-out. Aerobic exercise of course is most effective in this regard. Rebounding exercise on a miniature trampoline for only a few minutes several times a day has been shown to achieve huge benefits in health to sedentary people, and it has become abundantly clear that frequent light exercise alone, by its stimulating effect on the flow of lymph — the *milieu interieur* — is to be regarded as vital to the maintenance of health.

Cardiovascular efficiency

Kenneth Cooper's book *Aerobics* led probably millions of people to misunderstand just what cardiovascular fitness was. Cooper implied that the Training Effect and cardiovascular efficiency were one and the same — in other words you can't have one without the other. But as I discovered for myself over the past couple of years observing the effect of reducing my running activity almost to zero but keeping moderately active, on a diet mainly of fruit, my resting pulse increased only to 45 and my blood pressure not at all (110/65). My stamina is still good and I still never "catch" colds while working as long and hard as ever. Pritikin was right

— in health and longevity, diet is the most important factor. Maybe there are in the world millions of pairs of running shoes being worn out for nothing, or should I say millions of pairs of running shoes which could have lasted a lot longer. Be that as it may, for myself I have no regrets.

To clarify this point about cardiovascular efficiency, I shall quote Albert E. Carter from his book *The Miracles of Rebound Exercise* (1979): "Cooper's premise is that the answer is oxygen circulation to the cells. Granted, oxygen is necessary; but perhaps he was too close to the real answer to recognise it. Perhaps the real answer is efficient body fluid circulation to the cells. You see, any activity that would cause increased oxygen circulation would also cause increased fluid circulation. Therefore, as Aerobics was studied, all of the benefits appeared to be because of efficient oxygen consumption, when in fact, many of the benefits of the activity were a combination of better lymphatic circulation, better delivery of nutrients by the blood, more efficient oxygen utilization from the lungs, and better elimination and digestion because of more efficient body fluid circulation.

"Maximum cardiovascular efficiency can be achieved by rebounding aerobically five four-minute periods each day. Any longer than that is not going to improve heart efficiency noticeably.

"It makes no difference how much oxygen is available to cells if the right nutrients are not there. Even if oxygen and foodstuffs are readily available, with too many toxins, poisons or trash in the lymph fluid surrounding the cells and hampering proper cellular function, good health would not be likely.

"The body can't possibly have an overly efficient fluid circulation system. Efficient fluid circulation is synonymous with physical fitness."

Exercise and longevity

Dr De Lacy Evans, as already mentioned, noted that sedentary people as well as active people lived to a hundred years or more and that the common factor among centenarians was that they all ate sparingly.

As the three most dangerous components of the Western diet are fat, cholesterol and excess protein, and as Aerobic exercise achieves a large degree of protection against the effects of fat but not against cholesterol and excess protein, it is of the utmost importance for athletes to realize the benefits of physical fitness, although real, are not all-embracing, and that super-fitness does not necessarily mean super-health.

CHAPTER TWELVE

Dieting For Longevity

"We do not degenerate because we grow old, we grow old because we degenerate." — The Health Revolution

Walking through Rushcutters Bay Park, Sydney, with Nathan Pritikin one day during one of his lecture tours, I asked him, "If you avoid heart disease, cancer, and other diseases of degeneration, when and how will one eventually die?" and he replied, "When you are about 117, you will go to bed one night and go to sleep but not wake up in the morning. You will have died of old age." I pursued the subject: "But what will have changed inside the body during the night to cause the cessation of its functions?" to which question he could only reply that the body would cease to function because it was worn out . . .

But do tissues and organs wear out or are they gradually destroyed by processes which could possibly be avoided? Scientific opinion agrees that the human lifespan potential is about 120 years and some estimates go higher. These estimates are probably conservative because quite a number of people are known to have exceeded 110 years without making any special efforts at all to preserve themselves. Be that as it may, the consensus of opinion is that by taking reasonable care, the degeneration which constitutes the aging process can be slowed down so that old age is postponed.

Old age defined

Old age is a degenerative disease of the entire body, the progress of which is determined more by the degenerating factors in a person's lifestyle than by their chronological age.

Old age described

Everyone knows what old age looks like from the outside, but what changes occur inside the body? In his book *The Span of Life* Dr William Malisoff describes the atrophy and degeneration of every organ and tissue in the body that accompanies old age and the malfunctions which occur as a result. He says: "The system of organs is so thoroughly connected that all these changes have mutual repercussions. Thus too the liver, pancreas, spleen, kidneys, urinary organs, become atrophied, hardened and degenerated. The capsule of the kidney is thickened, the parenchyma hardened; the connective tissue scleroses and compresses tubules and glomeruli, impairing their action. The changes in the brain, in the spinal cord, in the nerves, are of a similar character.

"The description of the changes would fill many volumes. We can summarize that they fall into several classes: the atrophies, which have been commented on; the fibroses as replacements by fiber; pigmentations; metaplasias; hyperkeratoses, or skin changes and the like; renunciation of functions, as those of the germ cells and the instance of fat cells which no longer store fat."

Dr Arnold Lorand of Austria, in his book *Old Age Deferred* described old age as a condition in which there is a diminution of metabolism, i.e. the assimilation and conversion of food into energy, and is characterized by the abundant growth of connective tissue in vital organs, diminution of oxidation and increased auto-intoxication.

Dr Charles De Lacy Evans of England in his book *How to Prolong Life: An Enquiry into the Cause of Old Age and Natural Death,* written one hundred years ago, was more specific; he said: "The most marked feature in old age is that fibrinous, gelatinous and earthy deposit has taken place in the system; the latter being chiefly of phosphate and carbonate of lime, with small quantities of sulphate of lime, magnesia and traces of other earths." He added that the deposits occur in all tissues including the bones and blood vessels, which harden and reduce in caliber, and quoted a Doctor C. J. B. Williams who said: "The process is, therefore, to be viewed as almost entirely of a chemical nature, and as consisting of the concretion and accumulation of calcareous salts, phosphate and carbonate of lime in the debris of animal matter."

Dr De Lacy Evans went on to explain how the fibrinous, gelatinous substances were formed by the oxidation within the bloodstream and tissues of excessive albumin (protein), and how the earthy deposits were derived mainly from grain products and root and leafy vegetables and to a lesser extent from animal products.

Dr Evans tended to blame the formation of the fibrinous, gelatinous substance on the presence of oxygen, just as some biochemists do today with their 'free-radical' theory of aging. More pertinent to the argument, in the writer's opinion, is that if the diet is correct then neither the excess albumin nor the free-radicals will present themselves in the first place to improperly use the body's valuable oxygen.

Dr Arthur C. Giese, Professor of Biology Emeritus, Stanford University, in his book *Living With Our Sun's Ultraviolet Rays* says: "In our multi-cellular bodies some cells, such as those of the epidermal basal layer, continue to divide throughout life; others — for example nerve and muscle cells — differentiate and cease dividing at birth. Nevertheless, they continue to function for a lifetime, with gradually lessening activity and progressively filling with insoluble wastes and pigments."

As the tissues slowly acquire these characteristics of old-age their decline is further characterized by, and is measurable by, a corresponding decrease in enzyme levels and activity. On the other hand, animal tissue cells grown in cultures in the laboratory, properly cleansed and drained, do not degenerate in this fashion and may outlast the animal from which they originated many times over. It is held by some researchers (at least in theory) that in ideal circumstances immortality is possible. Other experiments with live animals fed on minimum rations showed improved health and a life extension of 50%-100% over that of unrestricted control animals on the same diet.

The longest-lived populations in the world are accepted generally to be the people of Hunza in northern Pakistan, Vilcabamba in Ecuador, and Georgia in Russia. An analysis of these peoples' living habits carried out under the auspices of the *National Geographic* in 1971 by Dr Alexander Leaf of New York provided a good reason why they outlived people of the Western world. The traditional diets of these long-lived (by our standards) people contained only half to two thirds the calories of the average American intake, about a quarter the amount of fat and half the protein. Their carbohydrate intake was about the same but was unprocessed instead of processed. As well, these people got more outdoor exercise and were less subject to stress than Americans.

In his book, Dr De Lacy Evans when reviewing a study of centenarians in England in the 19th Century said this: "On reviewing nearly 2000 reported cases of persons who lived more than a century, we generally find some peculiarity of diet or habits to account for their alleged longevity; we find some were living amongst all the luxuries life could afford, others in the most abject poverty — begging their bread; some were samples of symmetry and physique, others cripples; some drank large quantities of water, others little; some were total abstainers from alcoholic drinks, others drunkards; some smoked tobacco, others did not; some lived entirely on vegetables, others to a great extent on animal foods; some led active lives, others sedentary; some worked with their brain, others with their hands; some ate only one meal a day, others four or five; some few ate large quantities of food, others a small amount; in fact, we notice great divergence both in habits and diet, but in those cases where we have been able to obtain a reliable account of the diet, we find one *great cause* which accounts for the majority of cases of longevity, *moderation in the quantity of food*."

Thus perhaps the first rule in dieting for longevity is to eat sparingly, whatever the make-up of the diet. Even on a bad diet this rule will still permit better health and extended life because less wear and tear will have to be endured by the body.

So it becomes clear that 'old-age' occurs because we take into our bodies, mainly in food, harmful substances which overtax the digestive system, cause toxemia of the *milieu interieur*, overtax the eliminatory organs, and to a greater or lesser extent in the form of foreign compounds, gradually accumulate in the tissues and cells to increasingly impede their functions.

It follows then that old-age can be deferred by selecting foods which provide the best nutrition with the least digestive effort and the least amount of harmful residues, and consuming such foods in great moderation.

In Conclusion on Longevity

That "a man is as old as his arteries" was stated first by the 17th century physican, Thomas Sydenham. That "a man's arteries are as old as he makes them" was stated by Robert Bell, a 19th century physician. Perhaps we can proceed one step further to state the obvious: "The arteries and all the organs and tissues are as young as the cells of which they are made and the *milieu interieur* which sustains them."

Diet is not the only factor in longevity, of course, but it is by far the main one. The closer we can maintain the *milieu interieur* to an ideal condition, the less will be the wear and tear on our organs and the slower the accumulation of the fibrinous, gelatinous growths and calcareous mineral salts in our cells and tissues.

Think of all those little cells. Says Dr Edward J. Stiegbitz MS,

MD, FACP in his book *The Second Forty Years:* "Superficially, the answer is simple; intrinsically, extremely complex. Whether the cells themselves are, or are not, potentially immortal is largely beside the point. The essential fact is that continuance of such perpetual youth, as displayed by Carrel's chick heart cultures,* is absolutely dependent upon the maintenance of *an ideal environment.* Cultures must be aseptically transplanted to fresh media at frequent intervals or growth stops and the cells die, poisoned by the accumulating chemical debris of their living, and starved because their foodstuffs are used up. Contamination with even minute amounts of toxic substances or any inadequacy of any one of many nutritional requisites immediately interrupts the marvelous life stream. ***The quality of the cellular environment is the determining factor, whether the cells be growing in vitro in a test-tube, or in vivo, in the living and functioning organism.***"

Your body is a living and functioning organism and you want it to stay that way. We know what to do. We have discussed at great length the factors responsible for polluting the *milieu interieur* of the body and to eliminate them would appear to be easier said than done. Not everybody can arrange to live in a tropical Garden of Eden.

We can only do our best with what we have available, and the first step, wherever you live, is to cut down on the things that do the most harm. Eat as much as you can of your food raw. Cut out salt. Think of those little cells. Think of how clean your arteries will be, how comforting it will be never to worry about cancer. Each step you take will improve your well-being and increase your life-expectancy.

Think of fruit as sustaining food and not just an accessory adding color to the side-board, although it is admitted that much of the commercially-grown fruit available today looks a lot better

*Dr Alexis Carrel at the Rockefeller Institute, New York, in 1912 kept alive some cells taken from the heart tissue of an embryo chicken. Properly nourished and cleansed, the cell culture thrived and appeared to be immortal, at least until 1947 when the experiment was terminated.

than it tastes. Lack of taste means lack of nutrition and possibly at the same time the presence of insecticide traces. Quality is important, and you can't jazz up fruit like you can jazz up other foods to enhance its taste.

Do the best you can, remembering Dr De Lacy Evans' words of wisdom:

"There is, therefore, a simplicity, a reason, a wonderful philosophy in the first command given to man — Man may live entirely upon fruits in better health than the majority of mankind now enjoy. Good, sound, ripe fruits are never the cause of disease, but the vegetable acids, as we have before stated, lower the temperature of the body, decrease the process of combustion or oxidation — therefore the waste of the system — less sleep is required, activity is increased, fatigue or thirst is hardly experienced; still the body is well nourished, and as a comparatively small quantity of earthy salts are taken into the system, the cause of old age is in some degree removed, the effect is delayed, and life is prolonged to a period far beyond our 'threescore and ten'."

CHAPTER THIRTEEN

Learning The Hard Way

"The history of mankind is an immense sea of errors in which a few obscure truths may here and there be found."

C. de Beccaria

Bill Culverwell of Sydney went through fourteen years of unnecessary trauma and expense, of unnecessary suffering and fear, during which time, in and out of hospital, his life hung precariously in the balance. When first beset by the common circulatory problems of middle age, he was not unduly worried because he had faith in the vaunted powers of modern medicine, but as time went by he learned the hard way that his faith had been founded on an illusion. He learned that in the field of modern medicine the only things you can count on are the upsetting effects of drugs and the doctors' bills that accompany them. Then, at his lowest ebb, Bill found salvation with the Pritikin diet only to have it slip away in little over a year when arthritis began to cripple him.

Bill's story illustrates perfectly the pitfalls in matters of diet and medicine that can trap not only the unwary, but the wary as well. The story has a happy ending, thank goodness, and is told in a letter received just as our final chapters are being prepared for printing.

December 2, 1987

"In 1971 I was 54 years old and enjoyed playing squash for an hour or so regularly three times a week. I came off the court one day and mentioned to one of the fellows I had a burning sensation in the centre of my chest which made me think I had some sort of bronchial trouble. He said, ''It's not that, you should see your doctor as soon as possible.'' When I queried his reason for saying that he said that he was a doctor and repeated his advice.

I went to my family doctor that same night and was told I was suffering from hypertension and would need medication. In addition I was to have an ECG and a blood cholesterol test.

While awaiting the results of these tests some days later, I had my first heart attack — severe chest pains in the middle of the night which were relieved in about five minutes by a tablespoon of whisky that my doctor, over the phone, advised.

On my next visit to him, my doctor confirmed I was suffering from Cardiac Ischemia and that my days of competitive sport were over. I must continue with the blood-pressure tablets and do some exercises. Exercises? What was wrong with squash? I thought.

My first reaction was that I was now 'old' and that my life was approaching its end, and these thoughts were reinforced with two further, but less severe, angina attacks.

I tidied up my workshop, put away my hobbies,and quietly prepared for the approaching end. Today I can chuckle at those thoughts.

Well, I took my pills, carried out my exercises, believing implicitly all that the doctor said, and eventually a year later was taken off pills for a few months. This Utopian state was short-lived however, and soon I was back on the pills again. Twelve and a half years of pills of all sorts — round, square, large, white, yellow, green, and so on, with regular visits every three months to the doctor for blood pressure checks and more pills.

In January 1976, now aged 59, I was about to leave for work when I suffered my worst heart-attack, one that Anginine pills, the heart patients' first-aid kit, could not control. Living near a big hospital, my wife drove me there in five minutes where I recovered in Casualty while waiting for the absent staff to return. I was released a week later with a new pill added to my diet, and carried on as before save that a change in my job with the addition of overtime made exercising a late night chore, so that went by the board although I kept up my daily walking.

Three and a half years later, at age 63, my physical capacity had deteriorated so that the eight hour day became too arduous, walking up hills too difficult, and the doctor decided it was time for a coronary bypass operation. I took early retirement from work in August 1980, and entered hospital in January 1981 where a four-branch coronary bypass was performed, and after the sternum knitted, I was a rejuvenated man. I no longer needed Anginine pills to get up hills as fast as I liked. My spirits soared, this was Heaven. My only worry was, how long would it last? The medics would not give any opinion, but the hospital grape-vine said about five years.

Mine lasted only eight months before I was conscious of a definite down-turn in performance and in November I suffered a short-term stroke which lasted about six or seven minutes and I learned what paralysis was like — the leaden limbs, thickened tongue, loss of control of the right leg etc. While waiting for an appointment with the specialist I had six more but each one was to a lesser degree. 'T.I.A.' the medicos call it — temporary ischemic attack.

By March 1982 I was in worse condition than before the operation, with a pill dosage to suit. That marvellous life-saving operation had turned out to be just a very expensive band-aid, and I told them so. So back into hospital I went for more tests — angiograms, C.A.T. scans, Doppler machines etc. All showed the carotid arteries were 50% blocked, and the cranial syphon that feeds the brain was 80% blocked. My disease was making progress; where to next? I thought.

Further testing with ultra-sound and a medical committee of three doctors made a decision; the risks of bypassing the syphon outweighed the potential benefits, and to bypass the carotids without the syphon was also too risky because a worse blockage could ensue bringing on a full-scale stroke. I was put in the 'too hard' basket and sent home — no treatment, no advice.

March 1983 saw me back in hospital again with T.I.A. I was put on the Heparin drip and a week later was discharged with a new drug, Warfarin, to use. Like Heparin this is an anti-clotting drug and it is also the effective ingredient in Ratsak. On the way out I was referred to a kindly old doctor who explained to me all that one needed to know about the management of this drug, how it was essential to check the blood every six weeks, of the need to carry a special little red book with all the details of treatment, dosages, doctors' names, phone numbers etc. on my person at all times, in case of accident. I then asked him what the disease was that I had and he told me, Atherosclerosis — a term which until then had never been mentioned to me. He went on to describe how the plaque accumulated in the walls of the arteries until it eventually caused complete blockages; it was not known why it occurred, nor was there any cure for it. It was then I realized and had the doctor confirm, that all the thousands of pills I had taken over the last twelve years were never intended to treat the disease but merely to hide the symptoms while it progressed on its merry way!

And what was there after Warfarin? I sensed nothing, from the attitude of the doctors, and a friendly hospital Sister confirmed this.

I arrived home feeling rejected, dejected, and without hope. I felt I had been 'conned' and defrauded, and my implicit faith in the modern skills of doctors vanished on the spot. There seemed very little future, except possibly for one thing. During this last stay in hospital one day my usual hospital doctor on his daily rounds with two others, dallied a moment as the others moved on and said, "Why don't you eat less fat?" I was puzzled by this as I had always followed the Health Department's recommendations and was not overweight, so I asked 'How do you mean?'

and he replied, 'Less milk and dairy foods,' and turned on his heel to rejoin his confreres. So back home I pondered on this remark; could it be he was giving me a tip? A clue to improving my health? I decided he was!

My wife's cousin is a bibliophile, haunting bookshops, keen on unusual 'fringe' subjects. She bought me a copy of *The Pritikin Program of Diet and Exercise.* It read convincingly; even if only half true, it was worth a try, for was I not a 'drowning man' so to speak? Later on she bought me your *Health Revolution* which was written in terms much easier to understand. I read it from cover to cover.

At this time, July 1983, my physical capacity was very poor. My walks were puncutated with frequent stops due to intense intermittent claudication pains in hips and legs. I could not make the next street *downhill* without a rest. I went nowhere without my Anginine pills, and if I sat down for more than about forty minutes, say to watch television, I was beset with severe cramps in either one or both legs when I attempted to rise. Hands and feet were always cold. Between claudication, cramps and T.I.A. I could only visualize at best, my future in a wheelchair. But how soon?

In late July I went on the Pritikin diet and in ten days felt much brighter in spirit and I could work for longer periods. I walked up and down hills without pain or pills, it was fun, so I walked up and down hilly River Road 5½ kilometres to my friend's place and back again without a single pain. Was this the diet? Working so quickly?

I was all the time hungry, eating like a horse and at the same time losing weight at the rate of three pounds a week. Two weeks later I played men's doubles tennis with better players than myself and sweated, puffed, and ran hard for two hours straight, all without a pain. I was ecstatic! By the middle of September I ran in full strides down the hill where before I couldn't make one block, and continued on for 800 metres non-stop. I hadn't run that far for many years. But I had a touch of dizziness and it turned out it was due to my blood pressure pills — I didn't need them any more! After twelve and a half years with blood pressure 150/90 on pills I was down to 140/70 without them. All because of the Pritikin diet, it was hard to believe.

A year of exuberant living passed, I felt so well and was enjoying my tennis, sailing and snooker etc. and started preparing for the National Sailing Championships in January. This was in November 1984 and all of a sudden I noticed an annoying pain in the nape of my neck and minor pains in the left hip and right knee. After three or four days of this the pain was worse, so once again I went to the doctor.

In the next fortnight I kept eight medical appointments and was finally admitted to hospital for further tests including a bone scan; they were looking for cancer. During that fortnight, any neck movement increased the pain which had now moved upwards between the ears. Any attempt to lie down raised the level of pain and precluded any sleep. For fourteen nights I slept (?) sitting in a chair, by which time I was so exhausted and depressed, I felt that death was preferable, and I don't mind admitting it. Then the pain lessened, I was home again and able to sleep. I had lost fourteen pounds in weight. Throughout this period no diagnosis was given, and no pain-killers, but I had some physiotherapy which after four treatments I abandoned as useless. I then visited a chiropractor who gave me some relief and I began to feel hopeful. I had eight more visits and was wearing a special soft collar which gave me more comfort but I still had restricted neck movement.

In February and March of 1985 I was again being shuffled from one specialist to another without diagnosis or treatment and finally 'blew my top' and demanded something for the money they were taking. Action followed. I was told the problem was calcium dust from deterioriating bones getting in the joints, much as sand gets in a bearing, and the nerves were complaining. The knuckles in both my hands now had arthritic nodules, and in the mornings I could not close my fingers to the palms. Why should I get arthritis when I was eating a-la-Pritikin? I felt well, sailed my boat, walked every day, why arthritis:?

I referred to your *Health Revolution* and began a check on my eating habits — Weet Bix for breakfast with toast, pasta for lunch, etc. and decided that some 40% of my diet was wheat!

I promptly corrected all that, and following on what you said at one of your lectures I attended, turned largely to fresh fruit. Quickly the problems vanished. I now have no signs, no nodules, or any restrictions of movement that could be associated with the dreaded arthritis. Yet when I had asked the state's leading rheumatologist would a diet help me recover, he replied that all the research had indicated that diet was in no way connected with or had any effect on arthritis. But about six months ago I was happy to read a press statement by the same fellow that there was now evidence suggesting that one form at least of arthritis may respond to diet.

During this arthritis episode exercise was painful and walking was done with a limp but now, although free of restriction, my physical capacity had lessened, my lap time on my hilly circuit had increased from 29 minutes to 37 minutes and at times required an Anginine pill to keep going. Apparently atheroma flourishes while arthritis reigns, a la your story of Pope Paul. It took almost a year to recover my lost weight which is now static at 141 pounds but I still have not recovered my lost performance. I feel I should exercise more but my long bout with arthritis was followed by twisting my right leg and damaging some ligaments getting through the ceiling manhole last December, and they are still sensitive. I think I'll do as you suggest and abandon grain products altogether.

Early this year, I noticed a press item that the drug Hygroton had been removed from use in America because although it brought about a reduction in blood pressure, in the long term it reversed its effect, and furthermore it caused calcium loss in the bones. Also, being a diuretic, it reduces the amount of fluid in the body which presumably includes blood. As one doctor explained to me, the less fluid, the less work for the heart to do and the less blood pressure. Commonsense challenges this view because less fluid means thicker blood, therefore more pressure needed and more work for the heart.

Over a period of some twenty five years, I had developed a high regard for our old type 'family doctor' who prescribed my heart pills for the first ten years of my complaint until he retired at age 83. We had established a closer relationship than is normal between doctor and patient, so I visited him socially after I had started the diet and told him what wonderful things it was doing for me, of how it improved blood flow by reducing the fats in the blood. I was shocked by his reply. 'Oh,' he said, 'fats in the blood, that's been known about for years.' I bit my tongue on the obvious rejoinder, it was better to remain friends now. But here again I felt defrauded; I had not been given the best advice available, but sold a 'pig in a poke', and the doctors wonder why their credibility diminishes!

As a sign of the times, my wife told me only yesterday, that a friend had just been told by her doctor that she had high blood pressure. 'But,' he said, 'I won't give you pills, I want you to follow this diet.'

Ross, I set out to write you a letter but I feel it is now almost a book. I sincerely hope it doesn't bore you to tears, but how do you condense 17 years and 143 medical and hospital appointments for heart disease and arthritis alone, and still tell it properly?

Perhaps I sound bitter, but why didn't my doctor tell me what he knew instead of prescribing useless pills? Must our society have this medical hierarchy, the doctors, hospitals and chemists, which takes so much of our money and gives so little in return?

Be that as it may, with the knowledge I have acquired I have been able to assist some of the members of the sailing club with their problems, which is good, and incidentally, two weeks ago at age now 70, we got third place in the State Championships.

Yours faithfully,
Bill Culverwell."

CHAPTER FOURTEEN

In Conclusion

The present time marks the dawn of a new era in the evolutionary march of the human race. Out of the darkness of the ages where fear and superstition, greed and selfishness held their sway, there gradually comes the awakening of a higher consciousness and the cognizance of the great potentialities of man. To all progressive and unprejudiced thinkers it becomes clear that the universe is not at the mercy of blind forces, but governed by unchangeable laws; and that the phenomena of life and growth are the result of the wonderful and inimitable creative chemistry of Nature which unceasingly works towards perfection. The more closely and conscientiously we shall live in harmony with Nature's laws, the more we shall hasten the coming of a higher order of society characterized by the reign of intellect, universal peace and welfare of all.

—Otto Carque, 1925

The purpose of this book is four-fold, first to dispel the popular belief that grain products are health-giving foods, second to demonstrate that many other conventional ideas on nutrition are sadly in error, third to show that the cooking of food, alone, is a harmful transgression of Nature, and finally to point out that without so many dietary errors the human race could live according to God's rule that good health is the natural state of all living things.

An additional important message of course is that modern drug-orientated medicine is distinctly counter-productive to human health and constitutes probably the greatest example of "the blind leading the blind" one could ever imagine.

Specifically, the dietary information herein has been directed towards devotees of the Pritikin Program, people who have already made the effort to improve their diets and who may be to a greater or lesser extent, still making a lot of mistakes.

It is strongly suggested that health-conscious people should consider severely restricting grain products (cereals) together with lentils (beans), peas and nuts in their diets. I have presented some strong evidence against these food items and would point out that most of the evidence in their favor in the past has been based on false supposition. They are not required for their dietary fiber, they are not required to guard against protein deficiency, and their starch is not a better source of blood sugar than the natural sugars in fruit, as Nathan Pritikin thought them to be.

The only thing going for grain products is that they are satisfying and cheap, but considering their potential for causing harm they are poor value for money.

Paavo Airola, a nutritionist and health writer of note, who promoted cereals and nuts above all other foods, died of a heart attack at age 65. Michio Kushi, the leader of the world macrobiotic movement, which promotes the macrobiotic diet based on a high intake of cooked grains and other cooked food, looks much older than his years. That Nathan Pritikin survived 27 years after his diagnosis of severe coronary disease and lymphoma, gives great credit to his diet, but still he died of a severe blood disorder and failure of vital organs at age 69.

With the demolition of the arguments in support of grain products as a suitable mainstay for a healthy diet, and with the demolition of the arguments against fresh fruit, the fact emerges clearly that both the Pritikin diet and the Macrobiotic diet, for all their virtues, provide nutrition which is far from perfect. So far from perfect that one could liken changing to them from the

Western diet to jumping from the frying pan — if not into the fire — then at least into hot water.

But redemption is at hand — there is a happy ending. The Pritikin Center has recently announced that fruit is no longer restricted on the Pritikin diet. Good show! Now all they have to do is to restrict the cereals, or better still, give them to the birds.

Happy landings!

Index

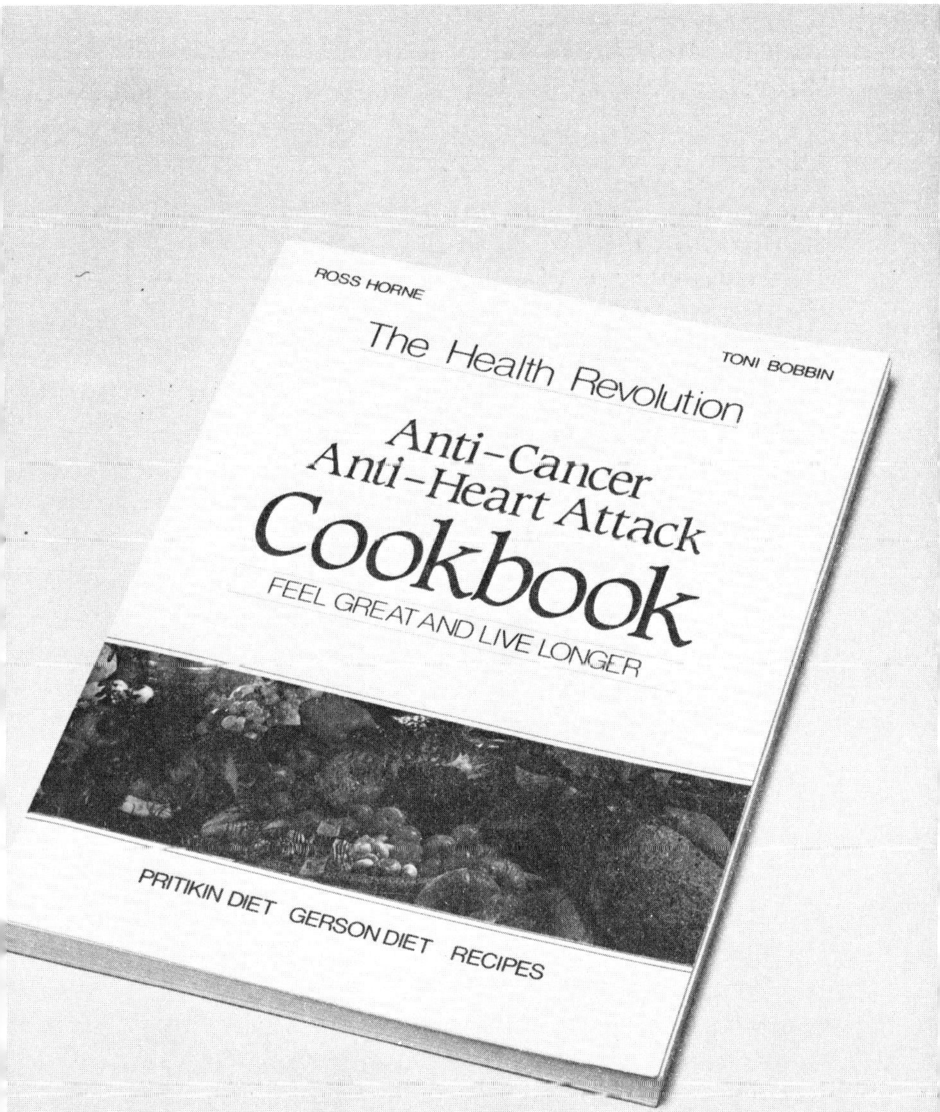
ROSS HORNE
The Health Revolution
TONI BOBBIN
Anti-Cancer
Anti-Heart Attack
Cookbook
FEEL GREAT AND LIVE LONGER
PRITIKIN DIET GERSON DIET RECIPES

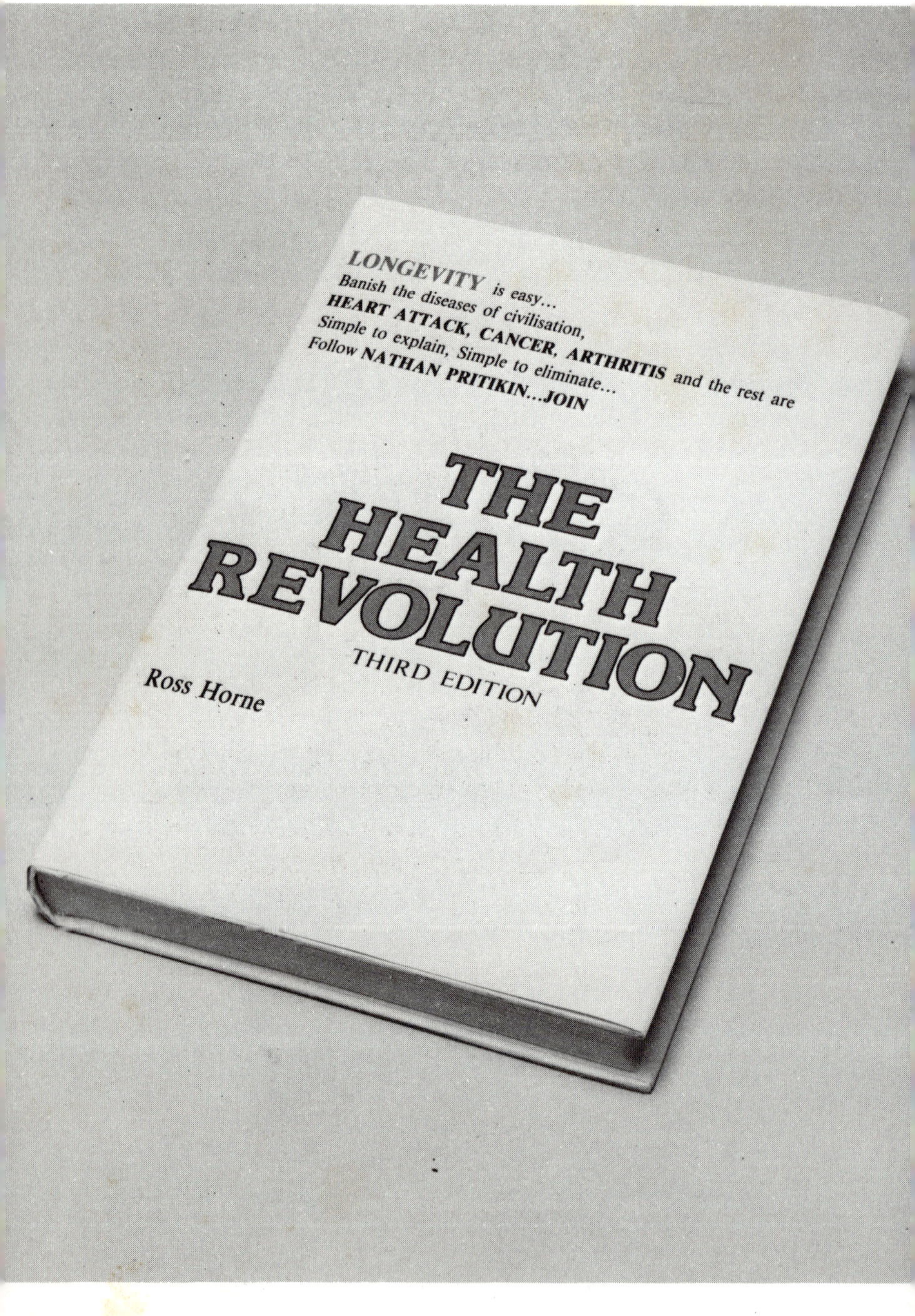
LONGEVITY is easy...
Banish the diseases of civilisation,
HEART ATTACK, CANCER, ARTHRITIS and the rest are
Simple to explain, Simple to eliminate...
Follow NATHAN PRITIKIN...JOIN
THE HEALTH REVOLUTION
THIRD EDITION
Ross Horne